To Ben,

Thank you so much for supporting me! Wishing you all of the best

△ Revée

My Sickled Cells

My Testimony of Resilience,
Hope & Faith

Revée Agyepong

TABLE OF CONTENTS

Dedication

I dedicate this book to my fellow sickle cell warriors, chronic illness champions and health homies.

Thank you for giving me a safe space to share my story and allowing me the privilege of advocating for you.

I hope this book encourages you to keep on moving forward because you never know what God has waiting for you. Your healing, cure or break through is around the corner.

Acknowledgment

This book is a product of nothing else but the love of God. Thank you, God, for my life and the many blessings and miracles You have granted me. God truly makes the impossible possible.

Thank you to my parents (Fred and Margaret Agyepong), siblings (Stephanie Amoah and Dimitri Agyepong) and brother-in-law (Edward Amoah) for the love and support you've shown me throughout my life. For lifting me up when I was down, for searching for hope when I was hopeless and for continually reminding me that I am loved and protected not only by you but by God. Thank you for the frequent book writing reminders, asking for updates and keeping me motivated throughout the writing process.

A special thank you to my sister Stephanie for being an advocate before I even knew what that was. Thank you for selflessly donating your stem cells to me. Transplant wouldn't have been possible without you.

A special thank you to my mom Margaret Agyepong for being my primary caregiver before, during and after transplant. Thank you for driving me to all of my appointments, reminding me to take my medications, cooking my meals, keeping things clean and putting up with my mood swings. Being a caregiver is not easy and I appreciate your hard work and sacrifice.

Thank you to my nieces (Gabrielle and Emma) and nephews (Malakai and Nico) for giving me a reason to keep on fighting. You guys gave me a reason to push through the hard times. Your warm hearts and joyful laugher is all I need.

Thank you to Pastor Emmanuel and Pastor Ibukun Adewusi for praying for me and pouring into my life. Thank you for the constant encouragement and reminding me of the plans God has for this book.

Thank you to my amazing editor Tumininu Agboola for helping me deliver the message God has laid on my heart. Thank you for dealing with my delays, forever changing timelines as well as keeping me on track and guiding me through this literary journey.

INTRODUCTION

Why hello friends, I'm so happy you decided to join me on this wild ride! Trust me you won't regret this decision. Let's dive right in, my name is Revée Agyepong and I am pretty much your typical 20 something year old woman with a massive medical record and a passion for helping others. When I say a massive medical record, I mean massive, no exaggeration, no fabrication, but simply massive. Sometimes when I look back at my life, I wonder how I made it through some of the things that I had to deal with from an early age. Trust me I will go through all of that in the coming chapters. So, a little bit about me, I am a daughter to two supportive parents, a sister to two siblings and an auntie which is by far my favourite title. I am a Registered Nurse with experience in Neonatal Intensive Care and Hematology. My passion for caring for others was really sparked by the nurses that took care of me throughout my life, so I knew I had to pay it forward.

Knowing that I brighten someone's day, puts a smile on my face. I am an extremely type A personality, in other words a control/organization freak, which probably isn't the best quality to have when you have a chronic illness that dictates your everyday life. I am generally a very positive and optimistic person but of course I'm human and have tough days too. Lastly, I am a believer, a believer in God as well as a believer that "I can do ALL things through Christ who strengthens me" (Philippians 4:13 NKJV). Oh yeah, I guess I should also mention that in November 2017 I had an allogeneic stem cell transplant to cure sickle cell anemia and it worked! I am officially sickle cell anemia free! I also became one of the first adults in Canada cured of sickle cell anemia! Pretty amazing that my little transplant made Canadian history and has been talked about worldwide.

Before we get started and dive into my journey, I want you to know the reasons WHY I wrote this book.

1. To inspire people to live by the guideline that anything is possible if you just dream it, believe it and work towards it.

2. To motivate people to advocate for what they need and be persistent about it.

3. To educate people about sickle cell disease and the realities of living with an invisible chronic illness.

4. To remind people that there is hope in every situation. Even when you can't see it. It's there.

5. To show people that it is okay to share your illness or struggles with people. Because no one can support you if they don't know what you are dealing with.

6. To remind people that they are experts. Despite what anyone might tell you. you know your body better than anyone else. Have confidence in yourself knowledge.

7. And last but not least to show people that they are not alone in their struggles.

So, if any of these reasons resonate with you, keep reading!

CHAPTER ONE

LET'S TALK SICKLE CELLS

I grew up in Edmonton, Alberta Canada. I was born and raised in the same house, which is always a shock to people. I lived there from birth to 27! When I was young my parents told me that I was a good kid but definitely as a baby cried more than my siblings. They figured that I was colicky, as some babies are but turns out I had a rare blood disorder that was rearing its ugly face. At the age two, I was diagnosed with a lifelong incurable genetic disorder called sickle cell disease. Here's a little bit about sickle cell anemia for those who haven't heard of it before or those that want a deeper understanding.

Sickle cell disease is characterized by its sickled/crescent moon shaped red blood cells. Rather than bouncy, flexible red blood cells (RBCs) that contains hemoglobin A, sickle cells are firm, rigid and love to stick together and contain hemoglobin S. It doesn't sound that bad, does it? They also only live for 10-20 days, whereas normal RBCs can live up to 120 days. Because these cells break down so quickly, and sometimes our bodies can't keep up with the demand for RBCs, individuals can become anemic which is a fancy way of saying low hemoglobin. These sticky sickle cells get stuck in smaller vessels in your body, potentially decreasing or in some cases completely obstructing blood flow. These blockages can occur in various areas of your body, for example bones, joints, and organs. Obstruction in blood flow to your body causes severe pain aka "pain crises". The pain is a combination of decreased blood flow, stretched vessels and sickled cells scraping the vessel walls. For me these pain crises could occur out of nowhere it seemed. The pain could start at a 5/10 and then escalate to a 10/10 within 30 minutes if it is not managed.

Areas of your body that are constantly being oxygen starved slowly stop working like they used to. Think of it like breaking a bone. After the first break, it generally heals well and, in some cases, you won't even remember it was ever broken, then after the second break the bone is less likely to go back to how it was before and as you continue to injure that same area after a while it just will not be the same. The same goes for sickle cells, if a bone, joint or organ is continually oxygen starved the result could be detrimental.

Long story short, this tiny genetic mutation has the potential to affect your entire body if you do not receive appropriate care. At times you might do everything right and still have multiple organ damage. Let's back track a little, I should probably mention how you get sickle cells; I promise it's not contagious! Thank goodness or I'd probably have no friends that did not already have it. Sickle cell disease is a genetic mutation that is passed through families, so to get the disease you would have to have to get a trait from both parents. If you have sickle cell disease or carry the trait it's a good idea to have your partner do a blood test called hemoglobinopathy or hemoglobin S screen. It's important to discuss your genotype with your partner and your physician to plan your pregnancy and understand all the options you have. Even if you don't think it runs in your family, it is still a good idea to get tested anyways.

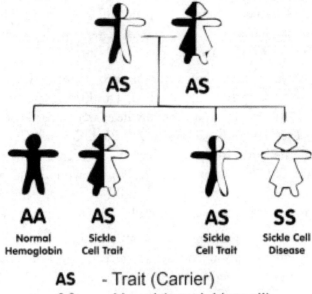

AS — Trait (Carrier)
AA — Usual (no sickle cell)
SS — Unusual (Sickle cell)

Sickle-Cell-and-Trait-Family-Tree-Square-300x300.png

Sickle cells is a very individual disease that affects everyone differently. Some people can go year after year without any issues while not on medication but then there are people that max out on all treatment options and still have issues and challenges. Everyone's experience with sickle cells is different. If you are reading this book and have sickle cell disease know that just because I have seen lots of complications in my lifetime, doesn't mean you will! Over the years I've experienced everything from crippling pain crises that left me in the hospital and completely bed ridden for days, a pulmonary embolism scare that had me clutching my chest and unable to take a breath. Hydroxyurea treatment that left me nauseous with stomach aches and blue fingernails. Red cell exchanges that left me exhausted but ultimately changed my life. Temporary femoral lines that had me crying as the surgeon tried to force it through my scarred vessels as the whole operating room stretcher shook. Implanted venous access device (IVAD) placement in my chest that left me scarred and feeling so insecure about my physical appearance. Gallstones that left me in debilitating pain for years until eventually my gallbladder had to be removed. Sickle cell retinopathy that led to peripheral vision damage requiring laser eye treatment. Hopelessness and dead ends that eventually led me to stem cell transplant.

Although I have been through a lot, I am so thankful it was spread out over 29 years or else I have no idea how I would have made it. I'll tell you a little bit about my family before we get into my early years. I am the youngest of three, I have an older sister named Stephanie who really has played the largest role in my sickle cell journey. She'd done everything for me from cuddling me when I was in pain, to being my hospital advocate when I couldn't speak for myself to eventually being my stem cell donor. Next meet my older brother Dimitri, he's best described as the life of the party. When I was down, bored or stuck in the house because of pain crises, Dimitri was always there to keep me company and make me laugh. My mom is Margaret and she's always been the caregiver of the house, I'd say she's best described by over feeding people when they come to the house. If you're in the mood for jokes and African food specifically Ghanaian my mom is your lady. Lastly is my dad Fred, he's the hardest worker of the family. My dad worked lots to ensure my family was well taken care of, and he's also gives the best advice when you need it most. Both of my parents were born and raised in Ghana (West Africa), and came to Canada as young adults for education and to start a new life abroad.

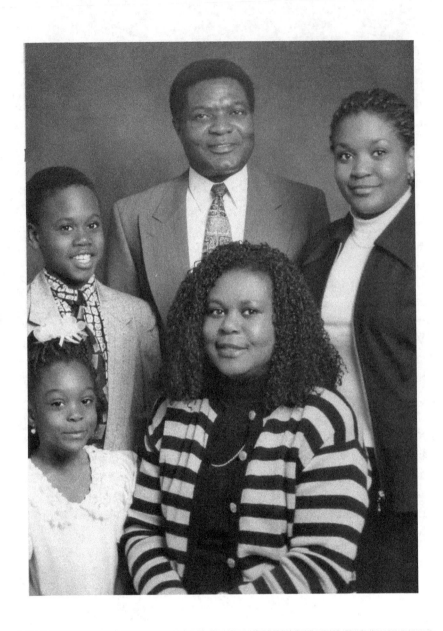

"Finding out that our child was diagnosed with Sickle Cell Disease was terrifying because in Ghana we saw how bad some people suffered with this disease. We worried if the doctor would know how to help our child because sickle cells wasn't seen frequently in North America"
- Fred & Margaret Agyepong (Parents).

CHAPTER TWO

GROWING UP SICKLED

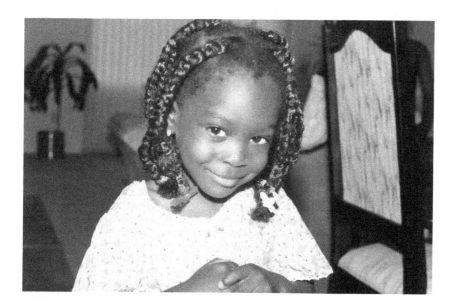

As a child I believed I had a pretty normal upbringing, the typical going to school during the week, weekday evenings were reserved for extracurricular activities and weekends for visits to relatives and relaxing. I spent most of my time inside, I enjoyed playing Polly Pockets and The Sims. I would play quietly for hours, to the point my parents would have to come down and remind me to eat. Sounds standard enough, but when I look back on my life, I realized that it was not normal. I vividly remember after recess being asked to line up and get ready to get back into the school. After running around for 15 minutes, I would stand in the recess line dizzy, nauseous, chest and back aching, heart pounding so loud I couldn't hear the chatter of my classmates around me. Apparently, that's not normal? I figured that was a completely normal response to recess and I believed it all of my elementary years. I never really told anyone because I didn't know it should be reported. I'd get back into my seat and rest my head on the desk exhausted, trying to catch my breath and silence my pounding heart. Another very normal experience I had was the nightmare I call "swimming". I know everyone reading this that has sickle cells can relate and those who do not are probably beyond confused, let me explain. Swimming is a normal activity for most people but for someone with sickle cells it can instantly throw your body into a pain crisis. The temperature swings that surround a swimming pool are hard on our bodies, in the water you're okay but the moment you get out, I remember being so cold that I was shivering. Cold makes your blood vessels constrict making it easier for sticky sickled cells to get stuck and become less effective at getting oxygen to every part of your body. The fear of drowning, and stress associated with wanting to be able to swim like the rest of the class probably didn't help my situation. I'd go home after the swimming field trip and go right to my bed because my body was already starting to ache. At a young age, I made a negative association with swimming so it's probably not a surprise that when I tried to take swimming lessons separate from school, I failed three times.

As I mentioned before, sickle cell disease is different for everyone, therefore each individual will have their own set of triggers. It's so important to know your triggers and find ways to avoid them, or work with them to give yourself the best possible outcomes. I had to learn this the hard way and end up in the hospital with pain crises before I realized something was a trigger. So, I'm hoping anyone who has not identified theirs takes some time to do so now.

Triggers

- Overexertion (due combination of dehydration and decreased oxygen)
- Cold (due to the narrowing of blood vessels)

- Flying (due to the high altitude and decrease oxygen)

- Emotional stress (due to the narrowing of the blood vessels)

- Dehydration (makes blood less viscous or 'thicker' and more prone to sticking)

I grew up not really understanding or knowing much about sickle cells, in all honesty I didn't even know the name. I just knew I had something wrong with me and had to stay in the hospital often is the phrase that elementary me would tell my friends at school after I missed a few days. I would miss large chunks of school here and there because of pain or infections. I remember being on antibiotics all the time, that it almost felt like a daily vitamin to me. I was never allowed to sleep over at friends' houses and back then I thought my parents were just being strict, when in reality they were scared I'd have a pain crisis overnight. Most of my pain crises happened between the hours of 7PM - 2AM, likely because after a long day of playing 7PM would be the time I'm finally winding down and my body realized that it was struggling to deliver oxygen to my body. I was fortunate enough to get a glimpse into playing sports, I played soccer and volleyball for a few years and cheerleading which was my personal favourite. Believe it or not, cheerleading was the hardest for me because of the intensive exercise and dance training - I only lasted one year. My coach would have us run laps around the gym followed by running up and down the stairs. By the end I was toast. One of the biggest things that I remember from my childhood was the feeling of missing out. Imagine that at the age 12, I already was experiencing FOMO (the fear of missing out). After a tough week in the hospital or when my body was aching but not quite a crisis yet, my parents would keep me inside resting to prevent any further issues. Which sounds like a smart idea but at the time I remember longingly looking out my bedroom window at the houses behind mine and hearing the screams and laughter of all of my block friends having fun without me. I know right, cue the sad violin. It was hard being too young to really understand why I had to stay in, thankfully Dimitri introduced me to The Sims and Stephanie to Polly Pockets which helped me keep busy during most of those lonely days.

Knowledge

Growing up my sister really saw how much this disease limited me and felt that likely more knowledge about it would provide me with ways to take care of myself. So, after a little convincing I decided that the first step to getting better was to accept that I had this condition. So, there was 12-year-old Revée taking control of her life. I figured what better place to find information than google. So, I asked my family exactly what the name of my condition was and they responded with "Sickle Cell Anemia," I took that info straight to google and slowly typed in s-i-c-k-l-e and then it popped right up into the search bar "sickle cell anemia," excited that I was finally doing something to get ahead of this disease I clicked it with a smile on my face. I remember having my notebook on my lap and so eager to get to it and start writing all of this life changing information about sickle cells. I can't remember the exact website I was led to but I do remember slowly working my way through the information. Starting with the importance of early diagnosis, signs and symptoms. As I read about the signs and symptoms, I felt a calmness and almost a happiness surrounding me as I realized that I was not alone. There are people all over the globe that were experiencing the exact same things I was. It's hard growing up with sickle cells and not knowing anyone else that was going through the exact same thing you were. It feels disempowering. I have an uncle who also has sickle cells but he was much older than me and lives in California, United States. Now I had the basics of what sickle cell anemia was and I had all of the symptoms of it, next was to learn about prevention.

To me this section was the most important because even at the young age of 12 I wanted to find a way to take care of myself so that I didn't end up in the hospital anymore. This section went over so many things I could do to avoid a sickle cell "pain crises" such as avoiding over exertion, extreme temperatures, high altitudes and staying hydrated. I felt like I hit the jackpot! I just learned how I was going to live a healthy pain free life. On to the next section - complications. This is where I started to raise an eyebrow and wonder if I was going to run into any of these issues. Some of the complications I read were stroke, organ/bone damage and blindness. My mind started racing when I realized that not only did sickle cells make me feel unwell it was also doing things to my body that I was unaware of. I tried to focus on the positive and just tell myself that at least I now have a better understanding of the disease and that it's better to know than to not know. Right? Then I approached the last section which stopped me dead in my tracks. This section was about life expectancy. Curiously, I read forward intrigued about what it would tell me. At the time I had no idea that all of these signs and symptoms and complications could affect your life expectancy. I figured that everyone lives a long healthy life and people only die from "old age". So, I continued reading, the site mentioned that without proper care many children don't live past age five. I didn't understand how this illness could kill a five-year-old.

Then I continued, my jaw dropped and my eyes swelled up with tears when I read the next sentence. It said that the average life expectancy for someone with sickle cells was 14 years old. I was in utter shock and confusion. I kept reading the same line over and over, confused how life expectancy could possibly be 14 years old, I was 12 years old therefore I only had two years left on earth. It felt like everything around me was spinning and couldn't catch my balance. I felt nauseous, my head hurt and my heart was beating so loud it was the only thing that I could hear. To be honest, I have no idea exactly what happened in the following hour, I must have completely gone into a state of shock or maybe I have just blocked it out because it was one of my most painful memories. Even now reliving that moment is very difficult. Feels like there's a lump in my throat and my eyes still swell up to this day. Because I vividly remember a memory so old and I can almost feel the panic that overcame me. I cried and cried and remember calling out to someone because of what I had just heard. My dad came and when I told him what happened he immediately closed the internet browser and told me not to believe everything that I read on the internet. Although that was supposed to be reassuring, it made me believe it more. He told me to trust in The Almighty Father and believe I would live a long life. When my sister returned from studying at school and told her, crying the entire time, I had taken her advice and learned more about sickle cells but what I learned was terrifying. She sat with me and consoled me and explained to me that life expectancy is an average and lots of people live much longer than that. Even with Stephanie's calming words, I still didn't feel calm at all. I could feel a fire burning inside me that no words could extinguish. I told her that I wanted to write a bucket list, that if I was going to die in two years, I would at least die happy. At first, she didn't seem on board with the plan but it seemed like after a few mins of silence she knew this is something that would make me happy. So, I grabbed a loose-leaf piece of paper and began writing. I didn't mention my secret bucket list to anyone other than my sister because I knew they wouldn't approve. I tucked it away in my desk drawer and referred back to it frequently so I didn't lose sight of what was important.

In the midst of my fear, confusion and disappointment I couldn't understand what I did to deserve this "curse". I grew up in a very religious home, we went to the Catholic Church on Sundays and went to Catholic Schools all through my life. I have always been a firm believer in God and was raised to understand that everything happens for a reason and nothing happens by mistake. So, I believed that, until the very day I found out what sickle cell anemia truly was. I couldn't wrap my head around the fact that "God did this to me". If everything happens for a reason and He is fully in control of my life then God intentionally designed me to live a short life filled with pain and suffering? That night I prayed the hardest I've ever prayed; it went along the lines of:

"Dear God, I don't know what I have done to deserve this curse. I will try my best to be a better person, daughter, sister and friend. I pray that you remove sickle cells from my body if that's even possible. Why me God why me?"

I prayed this over and over again as if I was chanting it and the more times, I said it the more likely God was to hear my prayer. I thought that my behaviour was directly linked to sickle cells, so I figured if I continued being a good person it would go away. My uncle told me that as he got older, he seemed to be "growing out" of sickle cells. At the time I didn't realize that the disease affects everyone differently and growing out of it really just meant the ability to manage it better as you age. I frequently asked God why me? Why did I have to have sickle cells? Why did I have to live a short life? Why am I in so much pain? Why am I in the hospital again? Something just wasn't adding up for me. At the time, I felt like I was a model child, student and friend. I always followed the rules (although I did talk more than necessary in class), I was always kind to others in fact I loved making others feel good, I always helped out around the house, but for some reason none of that was enough for God. I took a stand against this God and decided that I was no longer going to willingly go to church because I was tired of worshiping and praying when my case was hopeless. I figured I would just accept my early death sentence and live the little time I had left to the fullest.

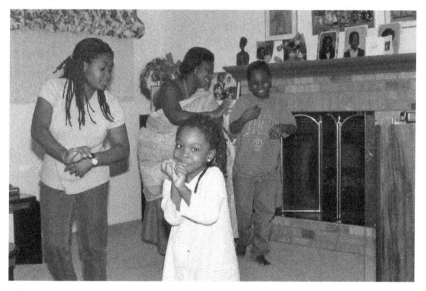

"When we were young, I knew my sister was different because she seemed to get sick very frequently. I found out that she had sickle cell disease when she was around 12, I felt helpless because I knew she was scared but there was nothing I could do to help"
- Dimitri (Brother).

CHAPTER THREE

LIVING ON BORROWED TIME

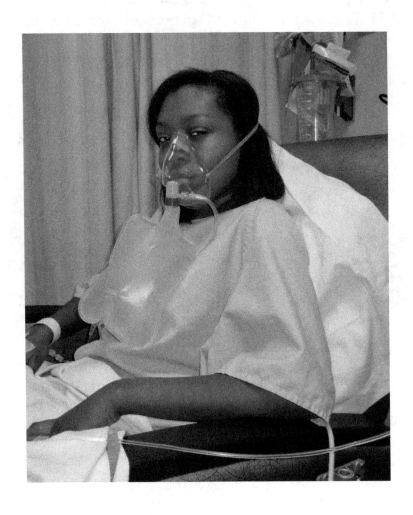

When my 14th birthday came and passed, I was confused. I have now made it a year past when I was expected to die. I wondered if there was a mistake on the website or if I was just going to be lucky enough to make it to my 18th or 21st birthday if we're being optimistic. Side note - at this point I had already accomplished everything on my bucket list so I was left with what to do now question. I wasn't really sure how to approach the extra time that I was allotted but my sister motivated me to dream. I found myself in grade 12 and actually looking towards a future outside of high school. I was always interested in nursing because throughout my many hospitals stays the nurses always make my stay better. I remember one hospital admission when I was about 16 years old, I was feeling scared and crying thinking that this could be the crisis that destroys my body once and for all. I found that every single admission I worried that I'd never make it out of the hospital. I had so much pain in my stomach, chest and legs and after days of aggressive narcotics, fluid and oxygen treatment I still didn't feel any better. The nurse sat on the edge of my bed rubbing my sore leg and reassured me that sometimes it takes more than a few days for the therapies to catch up to the pain to make me feel better. For some reason that ten minutes interaction made me feel safe in her hands and what I was experiencing was not abnormal. After countless beautiful moments with various nurses throughout the years I made my decision, I wanted to become a Registered Nurse.

Undergraduate School

I told my family about this new found revelation and they were thrilled at the idea that I was thinking about my future. That excitement seemed to die down slightly when my parents remembered that I have sickle cells and that nursing can be very stressful and hard on your body. I felt discouraged that my attempt to pay it forward was likely not going to be possible. Although everyone was skeptical, my sister took me to MacEwan University Faculty of Nursing open house. I remember being so excited, sitting in a class room bigger than I've ever seen, and listening to various students talk about what they loved about nursing and the many things they've learned. Little did I know that a year and a half later after the day I sat in that classroom I'd be receiving an acceptance letter to MacEwan University's 2011 Faculty of Nursing Winter intake.

Overjoyed that finally after applying on three separate occasions, upgrading two courses, and taking three university courses to boost my average I was accepted. I was a late acceptance so I only had two months before nursing school to submit all requested documentations, and fulfill the requirements. A combination of excitement that I was going to learn how to be a nurse plus the stress associated with worrying that I may not complete all of the requirements by the deadline plus working full time hours at a retail store over the holiday break to make money before school started plus sickle cell anemia equals one of the worst sickle cell crises I've ever had. My parents were away over the holidays, so my brother picked me up from the mall and dropped me at home, he had some plans of his own that night which meant that I had the house to myself to relax after working five shifts in a row. I got home, had something for dinner and then laid in my bed to recharge. That's when it hit me, the feeling that I've over exerted myself. I could feel my joints throbbing, my legs and arms heavy, my breathing laboured and my heart pounding in panic. I figured before this got out of hand, I should take the necessary steps to prevent a full-blown sickle cell crisis. So, I went downstairs, filled my water bottle, warmed up my heat pad, grabbed a bottle of painkillers and headed back to my room to wait out this storm.

Per chance my sister decided to pass by the evening and check on us, I told her that I wasn't feeling the best after work but had taken all of the necessary steps to prevent it from progressing. She wasn't buying it and insisted that I come and spend the night at her place. I was very opposed to this idea because I didn't want to be a burden to her. I figured that I'd be able to make it through the night on my own. Again, she said that it was more of her getting peace of mind knowing that she was close by if I needed anything. So, at that point I was convinced, I packed up my overnight bag and hopped into the car with her, if I had known what the next 24 hrs., were going to hold. I probably would have packed more stuff. When we got to her place, Stephanie, her husband Eddy and I watched a movie, I could still feel my body throbbing so it became hard to watch after a while. I opted for an early night and headed to the spare bedroom. For me, my go to with sickle cells was to lay in bed wrapped in blankets, rolled into a ball and wait out the storm. What felt like hours and hours went by and I was still wide awake just looking at the four walls that surrounded me, wondering why the pain was getting worse despite my efforts. Rolled up, in pain and whimpering is when Stephanie came through the door to come and check on me. She was in shock to see me in so much pain and wondered why I didn't call out to her for help. If only she knew that Revée's sickle cell rule #1 never ask for help because no one wants to be a burden. Steph said she thought she heard whimpering or crying and wanted to double check that she was just imagining it. At the point she found me, I was in so much pain I couldn't even sit up, let alone stand, I probably looked like a wet noodle. My body hurt so bad that any move I made would just amplify the pain by 10. Thankfully Eddy was there and strong enough to lift me up, I remember him and Stephanie slowly trying to lower me down the stairs and into the car. We rushed to the emergency room; Stephanie put me in a wheelchair to the triage while Eddy looked for parking.

The nurse asked me what was wrong in an attempt to triage and assess me, but I was in so much pain and out of breath that I could barely explain to her. My sister had to take over and explain to her what I have been experiencing, then after over an hour of waiting I was finally called. The one downside of sickle cells is that it's so "interesting" and not seen very often. When I was younger it felt almost like being treated like a lab rat. Every physician, fellow and resident wanted to sit in on assessment or ask additional questions about the condition. My personal favourite question was "how long have you had sickle cell anemia?" This is exactly what happened this time all the residents and doctors wanted to weigh in on my case when all I wanted was relief. My answer to their question was always "since birth, it's genetic." After the usual, three IV pokes, ECG, fluid boluses, oxygen via nasal cannula, IV narcotics with anti-nausea and hours of drifting in and out of sleep I still didn't feel any relief. That's when I knew this wasn't going to be a quick in and out, I was hoping for, I was going to be admitted. I was admitted and moved to the Hematology unit for over a week, I spent new year's in the hospital, lucky me. This was days away from me starting nursing school. Disappointed that sickle cells was yet again going to ruin another great thing in my life, I felt hopeless, that was until one nurse changed everything.

The sickle cell nurse came by my room and told me about the new treatment called red cell exchange. It was the highest form of sickle cell treatment available at this time and was working for some people. She explained that even though I am on Hydroxyurea it just wasn't working for me. Hydroxyurea was the gold standard for sickle cell medication at the time. It works by increasing fetal hemoglobin which is protective and does not sickle. Therefore, decreasing sickle cell crises, complications and disease progression. Starting this medication gave me hope for a bright future, however unfortunately this allure didn't last for very long as it stopped working for me. It turned my nails blue and gave me daily stomach pain that was almost unbearable. All while not keeping me out of the hospital. She explained that red cell exchange was essentially a high-powered blood transfusion where through a large bore needle in a deep vessel, about 2000 mls of donor blood will be given and the same volume removed. The machine works by withdrawing your blood, spinning out the sickle cells for disposal and then returning the rest of your cells back to you. This process is also called apheresis. It can be used to exchange various parts of your blood system but for me the target was to replace my sickle red blood cells with healthy donated red blood cells. The nurse drew diagrams to show me how the procedure would work and then even brought the large bore line that would be used, so I knew exactly what it looked like. The veins on my arms were assessed and because they are tiny, I was told that they would have to go in through my femoral vessel so my groin. She went over the risks and benefits, potential side effects and all. I was terrified but I knew that I had no other option but to go through with it.

The next morning my sister arrived bright and early to support me through this new procedure. I was wheeled away in a stretcher to the operating room, first step was the femoral line insertion.

Never being in an operating room before, so as you can imagine I was terrified, wondered why it was so cold and wished that a family member could have stayed in there with me. I thought it would be okay as long as they didn't touch anything? But apparently it didn't work like that. I was covered in a green barrier sheet and my right groin area exposed and cleaned with the coldest iodine solution. I forgot to mention that this is not done with any sedation you get a shot of a numbing medication right around the area they will be cutting into but other than that you are wide awake with eyes flickering under the barrier. The line insertion wasn't painful but you could definitely feel the pressure. I tried to just put my mind elsewhere and not think of what was happening around me, although that was next to impossible. I frequently would hear the nurse call out "are you doing, okay?" and I'd always answer yes even though my mind was racing and I wanted to jump right off the stretcher. Once they had the line in place, caps on the end, I was repositioned for an X-ray to ensure everything was where it was supposed to be. The doctor showed me my X-ray up on the big screen and pointed out where the line was and the surrounding structures. It was really cool but at the same time made me feel queasy thinking that there was something sticking out of my groin at this exact moment. From the OR I was taken to the Apheresis unit, really it was a tiny room with a few giant machines that I had never seen before and curtains to separate the patients.

The nurses on that unit were vibrant, positive and made me forget why I was really there. They set up machines that consisted of what looked like 101 levers to switch on, lines to attach, and snaps to clip. I listened to them verify my blood against my wrist band and hook me up, and for a moment I felt like I was in an episode of Grey's Anatomy. Eight bags of donor blood and two hours later, I was finally done. Excited that I had gotten through what everyone had said was the hard part, but little did I know that the worst part for me was actually going to be when the nurse pulled out the line and had to apply firm pressure for ten minutes! Trust me it's worse than it sounds, it left me in tears and I was then given the nickname "princess Revée" by the nurses. Since they had accessed such a large vessel I couldn't just get up and go home, I had to remain in bed for another three hours to ensure that the incision was completely clotted. After what felt like an eternity and one of the longest days ever, I was discharged from the hospital and on my way home to prepare for the next day which happened to be the first day of nursing school.

I was so excited to finally start nursing school, but there was definitely a part of me that felt some hesitation because of my current health. I'd frequently question if I was good enough, smart enough and healthy enough to be a nurse. I had to push through the negative self-talk and just chase after what I wanted most. I remember hobbling into new student orientation nervously, wondering if anyone would notice that I was "sick" and had treatment the day before. That stayed with me throughout nursing school and carried on through my adult life. At the time I had no idea but now I know that I didn't look sick and people who I considered friends and were close to me would go years before they realized my little secret. Nursing school wasn't easy on my body or my mind. The long days, late nights, high stress, girly drama, competitiveness and heavy course load was tough. But I pushed through, some weekends I'd secretly slip in and out of the hospital with a sickle cell crisis and then be back in class on Monday like nothing happened. I never wanted to use sickle cells as an excuse as to why I couldn't succeed. Clinicals were tough on my body, scaring me into feeling that maybe this full-time shift work was going to be tougher than I had anticipated. With my health frequently landing me in the hospital, and slowing me down my doubts and fears about dying young began to creep back into my life. Knowing that I was essentially living on borrowed time I was always scared to make plans too far into the future. I had lots of friends in relationships that would talk about their dream wedding, how many kids they wanted and which area of the suburbs they wanted to call home. But me I was scared to dream of those things and never really have the opportunity to experience them. At this time, it was crucial for me to have a good support system that could pick me up when I'm down. Your support system doesn't have to be only family, it can consist of close friends, coworkers and neighbours. Mine was a mixture of all of the above.

Nursing school wasn't all bad though, I made great lifelong friends, learned more than I thought my brain could hold and it was also during the time I met my first boyfriend. I did this all while battling a chronic illness that had me in and out of the hospital like clockwork. I would often find myself getting sickle cell crises as I approached exam time or final papers. For me any type of stress would cause crises for me, even if I was over excited it's possible, I could end up in crises. Fast forward four years to one of my proudest moments ever, my graduation. Finishing and passing my final preceptorship with flying colours made me feel like I was on top of the world. I was fortunate enough to get a preceptorship in the Neonatal Intensive Care Unit (NICU), which had become an area that interested me after my niece was born and spent three months there. I was fascinated with how the nurses would effortlessly soothe crying newborns, calculate tiny doses of medication, and react to emergency situations without even breaking a sweat. I didn't think I was smart enough or strong enough to be that kind of nurse so many suggested that for the sake of my body I should just go into community nursing which was also another one of my passions. I didn't like the idea of people around me thinking that I couldn't do something so I challenged myself to face my fear and I was successful. After an exhausting 12 weeks of absorbing information like a sponge and working my absolute hardest, it was over. I was officially a graduate nurse and the cherry on top was that I also interviewed for a position at the NICU and got it! This young warrior was fighting a battle that very few knew about, achieved her dreams and landed her dream job. I'm so thankful for everyone that continually pushed me to do better, be better and never give up on what I wanted. This is a mentality that stuck with me for life. Never give up.

CHAPTER FOUR

DATING WITH SICKLE CELLS

Despite the lows that sickle cells brought me it also brought some really great things. Through local Sickle Cell Foundations, I met so many people that all experienced and saw life the way I did. Sickle cells also helped me weed out the "for now friends" from the lifelong friends. A lot of people wanted nothing to do with my last-minute cancellations, bizarre excuses they didn't understand (e.g., swimming causing a crisis), appointments running into coffee date times or hospital hangouts. I wouldn't have been able to separate the good, from the great and build such amazing bonds with so many people. Nothing shows you a true friend more than someone who is willing to give up their New Year's Eve party plans to sit in a hospital bed with me and watch the fireworks on a tiny TV screen.

In the midst of my sickle cell struggles, I met my first serious boyfriend. Dating with sickle cells can be tough because you never really know when to share this "big bad secret with them". You don't want to share too early because it could scare them away before they even have a chance to see how great you are. But you also don't want to wait too long because then you might come off deceptive. You can only lie so many times about where you disappear to for half a day every eight weeks for red cell exchange or why you didn't answer their late-night call during a crisis. When is it the perfect time on your date to slide in, oh yea by the way "I have a chronic illness that dictates my everyday life?" Yeah, there's no perfect moment. So, I did what any young confused sickle cell warrior would do, I forced myself to nervously share my sickle secret before we made it official. I vividly remember sitting in the University Hospital cafeteria, laughing, joking and enjoying our break together when I decided this would be the best time. Why did I choose that random day in the cafeteria you might ask, well because I figured that we were in public so people generally manage their emotions better? I wasn't sure what exactly I was expecting him to say but all I knew was that I was terrified. He asked me why I didn't respond to his phone calls the previous night, I would usually use the excuse that I didn't see it, or I was studying and fell asleep early. So, in reply I said "I wasn't feeling too well," puzzled he looked at me probably thinking that I looked perfectly healthy to him. He curiously asked what was going on exactly, so then I just came out with it and said "well I have sickle cell anemia!" I figured he was going to ask me what that was or maybe he knew what it was and would be fearful of it. Instead, he looked deep in my eyes and said "oh yeah I thought so." Completely shocked and taken aback by his answer a million things went through my head, I wondered if maybe I looked sicklier than I thought, maybe he noticed the days I was in pain and tried to hide it or maybe my countless health lies have just caught up to me. So, I bravely asked him how he knew, and he said "well your eyes are yellow?" There it was, the trademark sickle cell sign that I've been branded with, regardless of how healthy you look or feel your eyes will always have a bit of a yellowish hue. This is called sclera icterus and as a result of your sickled cells short life span, when red blood cells die, they release a substance called bilirubin and the levels of bilirubin are much higher in sickle cell patients, thus causing a yellowish hue to eyes and sometimes skin (jaundice). I wasn't sure if I was relieved that he heard about sickle cells before or offended that with just a glance at me I was branded. To be honest to this day I still don't know how I feel about that response. Our conversation continued. He told me that he knew people with sickle cells that died from complications. His attempt at reassuring me about the disease made me feel uneasy thinking that the only thing he can associate with sickle cell anemia is death. Regardless of his current knowledge I made sure I taught him everything I knew about sickle cells in hopes to give him a more well-rounded outlook on the disease, because they look at me, I have sickle cells and I am doing well. Our friendship progressed into a relationship and at the time had no idea the effects that sickle cells really had on a relationship.

Although we were young and people would assume we didn't have many things to think about other than our university grades, parties and when our next date night would be, sickle cells added a whole other level to our relationship. It could change a light, playful day into a night ending with a crisis. I was generally very physically healthy during this time but I realize now that my mental health was not in a good place. Most days I could enjoy his company and others I required frequent reassurance that I was enough. I was confident in my abilities to do pretty much anything but was not confident in my body because I really had no control over it. All of my insecurities and fears came to life when about four months in I decided to invite him to one of my red cell exchanges so he could see this big procedure I go for every eight weeks and what it's all about. I believe he had class that day so he joined me briefly during the actual red cell exchange and then kept me company during the two-three hours of bed rest afterwards. It was nice having him there, it made me feel very accepted and that he really cared about my wellbeing. After the bed rest is finished, before you are discharged you are asked by the nurse to walk to the bathroom with assistance if needed because you're generally light headed to ensure that firstly you can pee and secondly the incision remains closed upon walking. So, like any other time I slowly sat up, dangled my feet at the edge of the bed, rose to my feet and began hobbling over to the bathroom. Thankful that I could pee and my incision remained closed, I returned to my bed to change out of my hospital gown and go home.

Later that night I asked him what his thoughts on my treatment were, of course he commented on the massive machine and the hilarious Apheresis nurse, but I was shocked when he mentioned blood on the back of my hospital gown. He explained that he didn't like seeing my blood and it made him feel uncomfortable because he was unsure if it was blood from the fresh wound, period blood or spilled iodine cleaning solution. I was overcome with anger because all though I asked for his opinion I was in no shape or form expecting to get that response. Yes, I was upset but I forgave him realizing that this was someone who has never been admitted to a hospital themselves nor visited any one in hospital prior to that day. I believe it was a combination of fear, a new experience and being overwhelmed. After a few great years together we ended up going our separate ways for reasons that may or may not have had anything to do with sickle cells. This isn't a cautionary tale to scare people with sickle cells out of dating but the disease definitely can take a toll on your relationships. What I learned from this relationship is that although people may seem ready to experience some things on your sickle cell journey with you, they are often not ready emotionally or even mentally. On the same token you can't choose when you have a crisis or what happens to you during a hospitalization or how your body will react to a treatment, so all you can choose is the company you will surround yourself with during those hard times. That goes for romantic relationships as well as friendships. Honestly, I am no relationship guru but I wouldn't suggest you introduce yourself with "Hi I'm _____ and I have [insert chronic illness here]." But you know what I mean.

Sickle cells may be a deterrent for some people but also peak others interest in you. After that relationship, I told myself I was going to be upfront about sickle cells with anyone I was interested in. This is when I met my next boyfriend, he had a huge heart, loved to crack jokes and go with the flow of life. We met in a super nontraditional way, yes people online we swiped right. After a few weeks of back-and-forth flirtatious banter, we finally went on a date and met in person. We went on our first date at Earls for dinner, I remember being beyond nervous about not being able to spot him in a crowded restaurant. We spent hours that evening laughing, getting to know each other and making memories. Our second date was an afternoon coffee date, we sat on the patio drinking our frozen drinks while the sun shone on us. It was there that he caught a glimpse of the bandage on my right chest and asked what happened. I realized that I only had two options, tell him the truth that I had just gotten an implanted port and have to explain what that is, why I need one etcetera. Or I could make something up and prolong the inevitable. So, I worked up all the courage that I had knowing that once I open this can of worms I could be bombarded with questions and this could potentially be our last date. I told him that it was called an "IVAD which stood for implanted venous access device," I continued on telling him that "it is used for high powered blood transfusions." I waited nervously not really sure what type of response I was going to get from him. He curiously asked me.... I went on to tell him that I was born with a rare blood disorder and this was the treatment I needed to stay healthy. He responded with a smile and then thanked me for being so open with him because he could tell how hard it was for me. At the end of the date, I had wondered if I told him too much or if I'd ever see him again. I know that my health can be intimidating and cause people to run. Instead, he walked me to my car, hugged me and said "text me when you get home". Just like that our relationship took off, date after date we grew closer and learned more about each other. Our relationship was full of laughter, support for each other and lots of love. I am so thankful that he came into my life when he did because I was about to climb a huge mountain and go through so many changes, which would have been difficult without his support and encouragement. Our adventures didn't last forever but he stuck by me through some of the hard times ahead.

CHAPTER FIVE

RUNNING OUT
OF OPTIONS

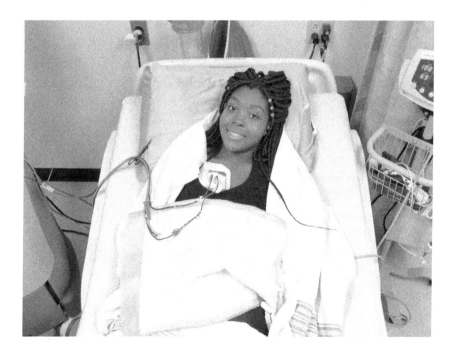

A s time went by my body became more and more used to red cell exchange, and it was no longer this life changing treatment but rather a form of maintaining my health. I continued to work full time 12 hrs. shifts in the Neonatal ICU, then walk downstairs to the Apheresis room after a night shift to get my treatment. It made for a long day but I was determined to maintain a normal life whilst still managing my disease. Only a few of my coworkers knew that I had sickle cells and they only knew because I made the decision to let some people in just in case something was ever to happen to me at work. I didn't want everyone to know for a few reasons.

1. Because I didn't want to be treated differently, in terms of receiving easier or less stressful patient assignments and be seen as less than everyone one else - there it is again my sickle insecurities at it again.

2. It would just give people some gossip to talk about but I knew that people knowing didn't automatically translate into support and love.

I laid low and pretended I was just as healthy as the rest, which actually worked for me for two years until December 7th, 2016. Oh yes, you know this is a significant date for me since I remembered the exact day. It was a regular semi busy day at work, I say semi busy because there was enough work to do so that you wouldn't be bored but not too much that you're running around the unit frazzled. I was happy that it was a chill day because the day before I wasn't feeling too well, I had actually considered calling in sick but I decided against it knowing that I just had to work three day shifts then I would be off for a few days. My body was feeling worn down, my head was pounding and I could feel my hip and wrist joints throbbing. I attributed it to standing on my feet all day and having lots to chart, not sickle cells at all related. At that point I had small sickle cell crises here or there, some worse than others but I prided myself on the fact that for five years I was able to manage them at home. On my drive home I remember talking to my sister, I was stressed about something in my personal life that was significant then but clearly insignificant now. She advised me to take it easy and rest tonight. So, when I got home I did just that, had a shower, had a warm meal, chatted with my parents about our day and then went to lie in bed. Then it began, the little joint throbbing pain had become so bad to manage with the strongest pain medications I could find. I say medications because I know I took two different kinds of pain medication in order to really get on top of it. I wouldn't recommend doing that unless advised by your doctor but at the time I felt there was no other option and I had to go to work the next day.

Hours went by and the pain remained and even amplified, the thought crossed my mind that I might have to go to the hospital but I put it out of my head immediately. My mom came to my room to check on me hoping to see that I was feeling much better than I told her earlier but unfortunately, I wasn't. My mom is the career of the family. She wants everyone to be well and if she can't do it on her own then she'll insist that we find a way to get well. I think she struggled with sickle cells as much as she wanted to take the pain away, she wasn't able to, she could get me medication, water, a heat pad but in the end, I could still have pain. So naturally it made sense that she didn't want to see me in pain any longer and wanted me to go to the hospital ASAP. She called out to my dad who was already in his pajamas at the time and he joined her at the foot of my bed scratching their heads and puzzled how this pain crisis was happening considering I had my red cell exchange treatment less than three weeks ago; trust me I was confused too. After a bit of convincing and my own fear and worry creeping into my mind, I found myself agreeing to go to the emergency. It wasn't until I had to get out of my bed that I realized how much pain I was in, my little joint pain which turned into throbbing has now become a full body sickle cell crisis. I was at the point, the pain I was in was less of a question about where I was in pain but more so where I couldn't feel pain and that was in my feet and hands. The rest of my body felt hot, angry and as if it was punishing me for not taking good care of it. The car ride felt much longer than the 16 minutes it generally takes me to get to work, and more of a bumpy ride than I can remember, partially because I was riding in the back seat and partially because with such intense pain I could feel every pothole, stretch of uneven pavement and time the brakes were pressed.

Finally, we arrived at the emergency and my mom put me in a wheelchair and rushed me in. We got to the triage and I could barely even talk. I was in so much pain. I was pulled around by the nurse and I breathlessly explained to her that I was having severe

9/10 pain all over my body, with a headache to match as well as one side of my lower lip was numb. She took my vitals and was astounded at a temperature 41.1 degree Celsius, heart rate 130 beats per minute while I sat in front of her slumped over (normal adult heart rate is 60-100 beats per minute) and a blood pressure that was almost double what my normal was. Let's just say after that I didn't have to wait much longer to get a bed. The nurse called my name and led myself and my entourage of family to a curtained off room where I'd call my resting place for the next few hours. After countless tests that all confirmed a very severe sickle cell crisis and narcotics that put me to sleep but didn't even touch the pain, I was admitted to the hematology unit. Honestly the rest of this hospitalization was a blur, it seemed all I remember is I was in excruciating pain that I haven't felt in a very long time. It scared me since I was already on red cell exchange every eight weeks which at the time was the highest level of treatment available for sickle cell patients in my area. At the time I had no idea but this hospitalization shook me and my family to the core and it became the first step towards my stem cell transplant journey.

Although my health was in jeopardy and declining at a rate that felt like the speed of light. I tried my best to remain hopeful and positive. A friend of mine who also had sickle cells told me that she was taking a chance and undergoing a stem cell transplant. She said that it was being done at the Alberta Children's Hospital in Calgary which was a city about three hours away from mine. At this point I didn't really know much about stem cell transplant; all I really knew was that it was considered the only cure for sickle cells. Knowing that someone that I knew was getting a transplant made me feel hopeful and that transplant wasn't necessarily this far-fetched idea that couldn't be achieved. Conveniently my annual appointment with my hematologist was around the corner. Prior to my appointment I researched stem cell transplant for sickle cells so I could discuss this during the appointment. I prepared and hoped that he'd say this was something I could get. But man was I wrong. As per usual, I strutted into the clinic waiting room with my normal Agyepong family entourage, consisting of my mom, dad and sister. Shortly after arriving we were called in by the hematology nurse. She was a kind, hilarious, vibrant Irish woman with a bit of an accent and a soft caring voice. I loved seeing her because despite my outrageous worries and thorough type A questions she always made me feel validated and understood. I briefly mentioned to her some of my concerns with my health and current treatment regime. Then I told her that I was planning on talking to my hematologist about stem cell transplant, she encouraged me to voice my concerns and be honest with him. So that's exactly what I did. My entourage and I walked into his room, while searching for chairs and making place for each of us to sit in the tiny office. We spoke about my concerns with my health and feeling as though my current red cell exchange treatment was being less and less effective as time went on. I explained to him that I was tired of taking these Iron Chelation drugs that made me nauseous and my stomach hurt. Then I boldly asked "what about stem cell transplant, is that an option for me?" The room was silent for a second and then my physician explained to myself and my family that stem cell transplant is a very risky procedure, that there wasn't an abundance of research done on long term side effects for sickle cell patients, that with age it becomes even more risky, it wasn't being done for adults in Canada, only pediatrics and lastly that there was some new gene therapy called CRISPR that would eventually be in clinical trials and a better option for me. CRISPR is essentially a technology that locates a specific part of your DNA, alters that DNA and potentially has the power to cure illness. Long story short, I got a big fat, well explained and thorough NO. I know he could tell that I was upset, but he was doing what he thought at the time would provide me the best outcome. He suggested that we increase my frequency of red cell exchange from eight weeks to seven weeks and see if that improves my health. As well as reducing my work hours from full time to part time in hopes that more time to rest would help the pain crises. It was a good thing and I knew that but at the time it didn't feel like it. At the time I felt defeated and that all my years of hard work and proving myself to my peers was all going to waste. I know that wasn't the case but at the time in the head space that I was in it felt like a reality.

Psychologist Referral

After my family finished talking with my hematologist, I was off to see the social worker. She was a tanned lady with dark brown hair and always had positive advice to give me. After I sat in her room and got comfy, she asked me how things were going. I told her that things were tough, with my health and it was beginning to affect my work life and ultimately my happiness. She handed me a card and it read "insight psychological," not knowing what that was. I looked at her confused and she asked me if I'd ever spoken to someone about how I was feeling. Even more confused I responded "yeah my family and now you?" She encouraged me to speak to a psychologist because it would be an objective person that could provide me with feedback, reassurance and teach me how to work through some of the feelings I was having. I thanked her for the card but the only thing that was going through my head was "she thinks I'm crazy." At the time I had no idea how valuable a psychologist really was, and I thought that only people with severe mental illnesses had to see psychologists. Forgive me for my naive and ignorant thoughts.

After coming home from the clinic, I battled with myself on this whole idea of seeing a psychologist. Eventually I came to my senses knowing that this would help me and not hurt me. I picked up the phone and booked my first appointment. I was told not to feel uncomfortable because lots of people see psychologists and it's completely normal. I didn't feel very normal because at this point the only people, I've ever heard of seeing a psychologist were people with diagnoses of mental illnesses. I figured that I was going to walk into that office as Revée Agyepong the girl with sickle cells and walk out as Revée Agyepong the girl with sickle cells and mental illness. I was terrified of having both a physical and mental illness so I kept pushing back the date of my appointment. Eventually despite me trying to dodge the inevitable I found my name being called out of the waiting room and following a lady who was my psychologist down a hallway. I awkwardly scanned the room looking for somewhere to sit, felt like I was in school again and trying to decide if I wanted to sit in-front of the teacher or further back. To my surprise when she asked me "tell me a little bit about yourself". There was an endless flow of words coming out of my mouth and I couldn't control it. I realized that there was a lot more going on in my head than I thought. Here I was thinking that all that was on my mind was the fact that I had sickle cells, when in reality it was that plus family, work, relationships and much more. By the end of the appointment, I was really happy that I went, I felt a weight lifted off my shoulders that I didn't even know I was carrying. I went to the receptionist, paid for my session and booked another appointment. Then over the next few months I developed a bond with my psychologist that turned hesitation into excitement to see her. I am beyond thankful for that referral, I truly believe I wouldn't have been able to cope with what was ahead of me if it wasn't for some of things I learned through my psychologist. My psychologist helped me cope with my reality and my sister refused to allow me to settle for that reality.

CHAPTER SIX

MY ADVOCATE

My sister has always been my built-in advocate. I was fortunate because most people with chronic illnesses are stuck to advocate for themselves all the time. I vividly remember being rushed to the emergency one night when I was in junior high school, crying in the back of the car holding my body in the fetal position. Typical sickle cell crisis had taken me by surprise and what I thought was a little ache at 10pm turned into a full blow multi system sickle cell crisis by midnight. I was with my mom, dad and sister slumped over in the emergency waiting room until I finally heard the nurse call 'Ra vee Ah guy a pong' used to my name being butchered I slowly got up and hobbled in pain towards the room she led me to. I got dressed and patiently waited for a doctor to come in, to my surprise not one, or two but three doctors came in within a 20 minutes span each of them asking me to repeat my symptoms. Frustrated, I said repeatedly my chest, back, arms and knees hurt. It was likely that none of these doctors had much experience with sickle cells and didn't realize that the key with treating sickle cells is to act fast. My family, also frustrated with all of the questions from the doctors and no action being taken, decided to go for a walk outside of my curtained off "room". To their surprise they saw all three of those doctors huddled around a computer screen intently reading a website with the heading of "treatment of sickle cell anemia" so we were right, they had no idea what they were doing. My family came back to the room and told me what they saw, as annoying as that was it was slightly humorous to see that my case was keeping them on their toes. So, my sister got up and said to the next doctor that passed by my room "she needs pain control, preferably morphine with gravol, IV fluids and oxygen". The doctor stopped dead in his tracks, got his pen out and began writing orders for that. It was as if he thought that's what he thought he was supposed to do but just wanted to get confirmation. At that moment I couldn't believe my eyes and was so thankful that my sister remembered exactly what they did for me every time and was able to vocalize it when I couldn't. That's just one of the many examples of how my sister always looked out for me and advocated for my health. It was her goal to keep me healthy that almost made me want to keep myself healthy because I knew it was important for the people around me.

"Over the years I saw the pain that Revée had been going through, the activities that she wanted to do, the opportunities that were missed, failed treatments and the friends that were lost. It hurt to see her unable to fulfill these dreams or aspirations. I felt like if there was anything at all that I could do to improve her quality of life I should at least try. Despite the constant questioning and doubt of others (maybe due to lack of knowledge) I was willing to donate my blood (stem cells), for the chance at a better quality of life for Revée, I should at least try. I truly believed that if that's all she needed to survive, grow, become stronger and fulfill God's plans was my stem cells, I was willing to be that vehicle" - Stephanie (Sister).

After all of this my sister saw how much I was struggling and made it her mission to figure out a better treatment option for me. And she did just that, weeks later Stephanie presented me and my family with an option, an option that I didn't even think was possible. She stood up in the living room and opened up a black binder called stem cell transplant, I skimmed the table of contents she created and it consisted of several articles of patients who have received stem cell transplant as an adult, as well as various studies and research done on the safety of this treatment. But what shocked me the most is when I flipped over to the last page and saw an email from the National Institute of Health that read:

"Good Afternoon Ms. Revée Agyepong,

Thank you for your interest in our bone marrow transplant protocol for sickle cell disease at the National Institute of Health (NIH). We have several transplant protocols here for Sickle Cell Disease, which include a Full-matched sibling transplant and half-matched (or haplo) transplant. The full-matched sibling has the highest success rate at this time (around 85%), while the haplo (half-matched) is about 50% success rate (they are currently changing some of this protocol to improve the success rate)."

It took a second for what I just read to really sink in. I was in tears when I realized what lengths my sister had gone to. I always knew she loved me and I always knew she cared but to do all of this research and contact them on my behalf. I was blown away. I've heard about stem cell transplant and the NIH before but I never in a million years thought that NIH would be willing to take me on as a patient. I tearfully continued to read the email:

"Before we bring any patients into the NIH, the physicians will need to review your medical records. Once we receive this medical information, if it is determined that you may be eligible for transplant, we will invite you for a screening visit here at the NIH. The patient is responsible for airfare and lodging during this screening visit. The records we need are listed below:

- *Hospital and emergency room discharge summaries from the past year*
- *Especially medical records that document any hospitalization for severe vaso-occlusive crisis/ acute chest syndrome, history of stroke, priapism, etcetera.*
- *Most recent office visit note from your primary hematologist also to include most recent lab results*
- *Current medication list and dosages*
- *HLA-typing results on you (patient) and your potential donors (your healthy siblings)*
- *ABO-blood typing on you (patient) and your potential donors (your healthy siblings)*

Please send all records by fax, secure mail, or email".

As a family we all moved through the checklist of required information smiling, knowing that things were about to change and finally for the better. We figured it should be easy considering my hematologist had a very open chart policy, he believed that as patients it was our right to have access to our own chart. It should be as simple as sending an email to his nurse and asking for the documents I needed, then just like that I could be on a plane to Maryland, United States. It was all so exciting until I wasn't. My quick and easy thoughts of collecting all of this information then flying down to Maryland to be cured came to a screeching halt when I realized there were still barriers. I was on the phone and emailing my hematologists nurse on a daily basis asking for information, advice and approval. She was very willing and forthcoming with all of the information I needed, which made me feel as if I had her support. Then the next step on my long list was HLA testing myself and my siblings which was as simple as going to the lab and getting blood test done. Unfortunately, it wasn't as simple as I thought, what I soon found out from an angry transplant coordinator was that this test was very expensive to be done and it had to be done under the name of a hematologist not a family doctor that I had asked to write me a requisition for it. But really how would I know? So, then this is where things got messy. Essentially, I needed my hematologist to be the one to write the requisition, meaning that I would have to tell him what my plans were. I was afraid to tell him because I knew that once my secret was out, he had the opportunity to say no or potentially not support it. I also knew that to get another appointment with him on such short notice would be next to impossible. He mentioned at my last appointment what his thoughts on transplant were so I knew this was going to be tough. But I went for it anyways, they do say if you want something you have to go for it. So that is exactly what I decided to do!

CHAPTER SEVEN

A LIGHT IN THE DISTANCE

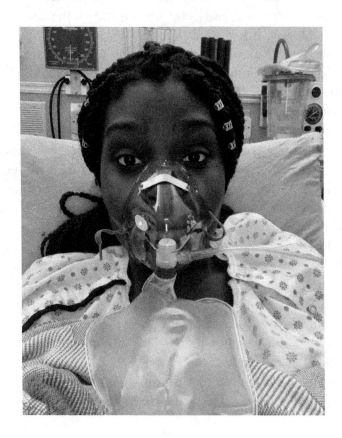

I was so stressed out during that time, guess what happened, in my midst of trying to change my life and adjusting to a new work schedule, my body decided I needed to take a break. My body told me this in the clearest way it could, and that was in the form of a sickle cell crisis. Lucky me. Of course, it wouldn't be a little kick in the butt crisis that just kept me home medicating, drinking fluids and resting on my day off. It had to be the "Hey Revée I need hospital attention" kind. So, that's exactly where I ended up, in the hospital. From the emergency room hustle and bustle to an admission to my home unit 5F4 Hematology. As much as I hated that place, it provided me with a sense of security, safety and weirdly enough home. So, I laid in my hospital bed looking up at the ceiling feeling alone but not, feeling sad but not and feeling in so much pain with no improvement. By chance my roommate was an older lady with a type of bone cancer that was waiting for a match so that she could have a bone marrow transplant. Crazy the chances that she would be my roommate. When neither of us had any visitors we would chat, I found comfort in the fact that we were both waiting for the same thing. Although she was already on the donor waiting list and I haven't even gotten HLA tested nor was I even sure if I was ever going to, it was nice to feel like someone else knew how I felt. Her symptoms were very different from mine in some ways but then very similar at the same time. Maybe God made us roommates so that neither of us felt alone, I'm really not sure but whatever the reasoning was, I was happy that it happened. This hospital stay was different for me, different in the sense that usually I would get pain relief right away but that wasn't the case. After days and days of laying in my bed and trying to take walks when I could, I still was experiencing 7/10 pain.

I remember having a needle in the back of my right arm into the fat tissue. This was where I would get my morphine pushes and then had another one on the back of my left arm where I would get my Gravol because these intense pain medications had the power to make me throw up instantly. After a while it became a routine, the nurse would come and check on me, ask me how I was feeling, I would respond with still in pain and she would ask me to rate it on a scale of 1-10, it was usually rated at 5-7 then she would leave and return to my room with a syringe of Dilaudid and one of Gravol. Then she'd check back in an hour to see if there had been any changes, I'd say not really and she'd reassure me that I should give it more time and see what happens and I would hopefully agree with her. Then I'd go back to sleep until the next time she would check on me. That was pretty much my routine over and over again. That was until it was broken and I was surprised by an unexpected visitor. It was my hematologist; he was notified by his nurse because by chance she called me while I was in the hospital. He was shocked that I had been in the hospital for 3 days at the time and no one had told him sooner. He asked how I was feeling and what exactly was going on. I explained to him the extremely deep throbbing that I felt in pretty much all of my joints but the most in my hips that it was difficult to walk. He looked at me attentively and with a deep thought look. I could tell that he was concerned and looking for an answer for me. But his response was expected. He looked at me and asked "are you serious about bone marrow transplant?" I quickly responded "I really am". Maybe shocked and concerned about my confidence in it. So, he asked if I had looked into the risks, I told him that I did and I was aware of how risky it was but I was tired of living my life like this any longer. It felt like every year even sometimes every month I would find out that something else was happening in my body. It felt as if the path that I was heading on wasn't going upwards; rather I felt like I was on a downwards spiral. After hearing all of this he told me to call his nurse tomorrow and book a quick appointment where he would go over more about stem cell transplant. I was so excited and couldn't believe what had just happened. So, the next day I did just that and I was booked to see him in about 2 weeks. Knowing that there could potentially be an end to all of this made it a lot easier for me to lay in the hospital bed in pain for the next 3 days until I was finally discharged. Side notes the in-house hematologist pretty much told me that the only reason I had pain was because it was cold outside and I didn't drink enough water. Which is probably one of the most belittling and offensive things you could say to a sickle cell patient. Yes, I am well aware of extreme temperatures and dehydration being potential triggers, however it's not the patient's fault that they are in pain. Everyone's body reacts differently to these triggers. Anyways despite her ignorance I just needed her for one thing and that was to write my discharge summary, prescriptions, and get me outta there!

Once discharged I spent the next week at home in bed still recovering. That is the one thing about sickle cells that I think people forget, just because you're discharged doesn't necessarily mean you're better. It means the hospital has stabilized you to a point that you can manage the rest at home. The following week I went to my hematologists office and he provided me with some additional information about transplant as promised. Then he told me that he contacted the Calgary bone marrow transplant team and they will handle my HLA testing that I have been fighting to get done. He told me to expect a phone call from them within the next two weeks. They called me the next day! On the phone I spoke to an intake coordinator that explained that HLA testing didn't mean that I was getting a transplant but rather it was only a test to see if I had a sibling match and if I didn't then we couldn't go any further in this process. The current protocol indicated that they were only able to go forward with a sibling match. I was told that there is only a 25% chance that you'll have a match in your family and then a 14% chance that the match wouldn't have sickle cells. So, the odds were most definitely not in my favour. Stephanie, Dimitri and myself all got our HLA tissue matching tests done, and then the waiting began.

Vacation

What better way to wait for news other than on vacation? My boyfriend at the time and I booked a trip to Los Angeles, which has always been one of my favourite destinations. It could be because I have no shortage of family on both sides of the family there, or maybe the perfect weather had me hooked. We rented a place that was in the heart of sunset Blvd., every morning we woke up to a backyard deck that had the view of the LA skyline. We got back from LA feeling great and so thankful that I didn't have health issues while away.

No Match

After being home for a few days I received a phone call from the transplant coordinator, I was excited because I knew what this could mean! Turns out it didn't mean what I thought it meant. The phone call was her telling me that my brother's test came back and unfortunately, he was not a match. I felt heartbroken and discouraged. How could he not be a match? Before we did the HLA typing, we were told that the best matches are generally closer in age and male donors are better because pregnancy and childbirth can make women form antibodies that they might not have normally. My brother fit the description for the perfect donor but surprisingly he wasn't. A few days after I got the news from the transplant coordinator my brother knocked on my door, and sheepishly took one step into the room, only one. And stood by my dresser then told me that he received his results and he unfortunately wasn't a match. I can't remember what my response was exactly but I knew it would have been limited to a few words. I was so upset that my chance of a stem cell transplant was pretty much out the door, with my sister already having two kids I knew that there was no way she could be a match. I remember feeling angry, not angry with him but angry with the situation. It was hard to feel so excited and hopeful of the possibility of a healthier life and then have it taken away. No one really understood how sad I was and how hard it was for me but really how would they?

CHAPTER EIGHT

A PERFECT MATCH

About a week after I returned from vacation, I received a call from my sister and she was crying. Confused and waiting for her to actually say something I sat in my bed holding the phone. She then said "REVÉE I AM A PERFECT MATCH". It took me a second to realize what she was saying because I had already put it out of my head that she would be a match. Then it hit me and the tears began falling and never stopped. I ran upstairs to my mom's room where she was laying in her bed. She looked at me with a concerned look probably wondering what the heck was going on that I'd be so frantic and crying. I put the phone on speaker and asked my sister to repeat what she said. Then again, she said "REVÉE AND I ARE A 10 OUT OF 10 PERFECT MATCH!" My mom also started crying and we sat there in her room speechless. My sister still on the phone said she couldn't even stay at work staring at her screen for the rest of the day so she packed up and left. Oh, I forgot to add that today May 1, 2017 was my sister's birthday. My mom and I excitedly called my dad to tell him the good news and then afterwards called my brother. Both of their reactions consisted of shock, laughter and pure joy! This meant that transplant was becoming a reality.

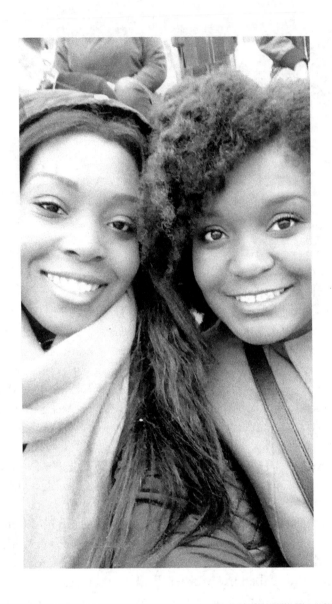

"The day I found out I was a perfect match; I was filled with shock and excitement. I was filled with fairytale thoughts of what her life could be like if everything went as planned. Then on the other hand I was like oh shoot, this makes it all real and what if it doesn't go as we hoped?" - Stephanie (Sister)

Process

Then we were on to the next step. Before we knew it my mom, dad, sister, brother-in-law and kids were in two cars, driving three hours to Calgary, Alberta for my first appointment at the Tom Baker Cancer Centre. I was so excited but at the same time so terrified. I didn't even realize it was possible to experience two extreme opposite emotions at the same time. Once we slowly found our way to the bone marrow transplant clinic area. We were met by a transplant coordinator with an inviting smile on her face that made me feel instantly comfortable with her. She led us into a tiny room that thankfully had enough chairs for me and my entourage. Shortly after we walked in, we were joined by a vibrant doctor, who introduced himself and asked for all of our names. After we all became comfortable and well acquainted the first question he asked was "so what do you know about stem cell transplant?" My sister and I looked at each other confidently knowing that we both have studied everything on stem cell transplant for weeks on end. He was shocked by the amount of research I had done. Knowing that I was a nurse and my family and I had a grasp on what stem cell transplant was, my doctor explained everything in detail. I showed him the three-page document typed into an excel sheet that was our family question sheet. Yes, we are a little dramatic but some would call us thorough rather.

Our sheet was divided into general questions, Revée specific, and questions for the social worker. After about a two-hour meeting with the doctor that felt like information overload, just when I thought I knew everything he just times it by ten. After the doctor left, we relocated to another room with the nurse and she went over the logistics of the whole process. Appointments and exams that needed to be done prior, what appointments would be in Calgary, how to touch base with the social worker about accommodations but of course the most important thing we discussed was, what's next if I said yes to transplant. That was the million-dollar question, was I ready? Was I brave enough? Was I really that tired of sickle cells? Was I willing to risk my life for a chance at a better life? That last question was the one that really scared me the most because I knew I wanted to be cured but I wasn't sure if a chance was better than the life I currently had. I would sit there wondering if my life was really that horrible that I would put my life on the line and risk death for a better life. I knew this wasn't a decision that I could make on the spot so I grabbed the consent papers, packed them into my clipboard and my family and I headed out. We thanked the nurse for all of the time she had spent explaining and clarifying things for us. She gave me her office phone number and office hours so that if any questions came up while I made a decision, she'd just be one call away. I appreciated her care in compassion during this time.

We left that appointment excited, hopeful and with a huge decision on my shoulders. Although I desperately wanted a transplant, I realized early on that the outcome is great but the potential adverse effects of chemotherapy, total body irradiation and transplant in general were even greater. Some of the scariest are GVHD (graft vs host disease which is when the donor cells try to reject your body resulting in organ damage or even death) infertility/early menopause, secondary cancers, cataracts, organ changes, thinning bones, joint changes, thyroid problems, trouble fighting infections and memory problems. In my mind since I was already blessed with sickle cells, so who says I wouldn't be so blessed to also get every single adverse effect? Yes, this is a super negative way of thinking but at the time I felt as if I was given the worst hand of cards. On the car ride home, I remember my head being all over the place, we stopped at Red Deer and had lunch then continued on our way. As I sat there in the car, mind racing, I realized that the slight pain and aching I felt earlier this morning that I attributed to simply being nervous about the appointment, was becoming more prominent, more intense, more sickle cell like. I told my parents that I could feel the pain getting worse and worse with every bump on the road. My dad is someone who tries to maintain composure in any situation, but I noticed from the back, my under the speed limit driving dad was going 10km/hr above the speed limit in hopes to get me back to Edmonton as quickly as possible. My dad was usually the one that you ask for a ride somewhere when you wanted to dottle and take the scenic route. My mom is the person who you asked from a ride when you're late for something, because you know she'll get you there on time, if not early. So, I was shocked to see my dad speeding, he went from 10 over to about 20 km/hr but that didn't feel fast enough. It's about an hour and half between Edmonton and Red Deer but when you're in 10/10 pain nothing feels fast enough. I spend the night in the emergency department getting the usual oxygen, fluids and pain medications. As I mentioned before, a trigger for me was emotional stress and this was a classic example of my emotions starting a chain reaction inside my body. This experience added fuel to the fire that has already been burning inside me, the fire that was to get cured.

I knew it wouldn't be an easy decision to make because there was ultimately no right or wrong answer. It was going to be based on preference, my preference. But what was my preference? On one hand I knew that the way my health had been declining the previous year wasn't leaving me feeling as if things would miraculously turn around and I would feel good again. On the other hand, there were supposedly newer and safer methods to cure sickle cells in the preliminary research steps. Then there were also the issues with fertility that transplant could cause, and I wasn't overly ready to give up my chances at having my own family one day. I expressed my fertility concerns with my transplant nurse and she happily took the time to follow up with the transplant physician and radiation oncology to voice my concerns and then provide me with answers. In her email response to me she forwarded me what the physicians had said and attached a few documents with charts on it that indicated what the potential of ovarian damage would be based off of my dose of radiation. It seemed simple enough with my 300 centigrade of radiation I wouldn't go into ovarian failure which seemed fair enough and put my mind slightly at ease. Clearly not for long enough because in two weeks' time I was calling her back asking her for more information on the chance of error that these numbers wouldn't be correct. So, she set up a virtual meeting with the radiation oncology team that could provide me with more in-depth information. I was so grateful for her at this time because she really did serve as a bridge between my uncertainty and feeling comfortable.

With all of these options and the what ifs on my shoulders I was full of chaos on the inside and tried to maintain my composure on the outside. I did what anyone would do when they are trying to make a huge decision, I made a pros and cons list.

PROS	CONS
I get cured	Fertility uncertainty
	Graft versus host disease
	It might not work
	I could die

As unbalanced as my pros and cons list looked. I realized it wasn't about how many pros or cons I had on either side of the chart. What really mattered was the weight of the one pro, I get cured. I never in a million years imagined a life without sickle cells but there it was looking right at me. I could potentially live a long life; I could do all of the things that I was never allowed to do or had to restrict myself from doing. I prayed day in and day out just waiting to hear from God. Then there it was, it hit me like a ton of bricks. I wouldn't have made it this far if this wasn't already God's plan for me, my sister wouldn't have gotten me accepted into the NIH trial, my hematologist wouldn't have agreed and referred me to the Tom Baker Cancer Centre and I wouldn't have had a 10/10 sibling match. So, there it was, I had my answer. I knew God would carry me through so I was going to get a stem cell transplant no matter what it might cost me!

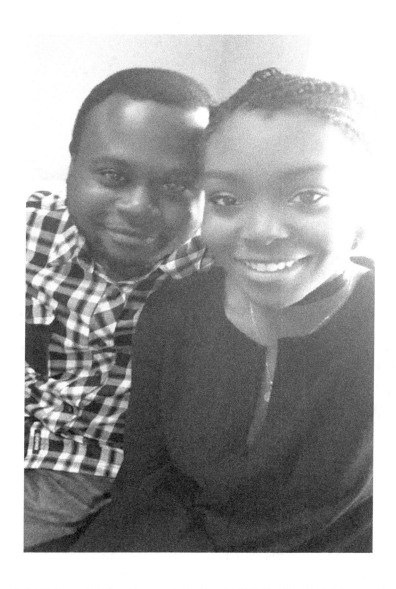

"When I found out that she was going for transplant I was scared and confused at the same time. But once I took the time to research, I felt better about it. Still nervous but I knew my sister could do it" - Dimitri (brother).

CHAPTER NINE

FERTILITY

From the moment I said yes, my life became a whirlwind, I was swept up into this world of stem cell transplant. It was as scary as it was exciting. The first priority on my mind, surprise surprise was getting a referral to a fertility clinic to learn more about freezing my eggs. I had a few friends that have had IVF and have shared their experiences with me so it made me feel like this whole egg banking and turkey basting world was a little less foreign.

Egg Freezing

My first appointment at the fertility clinic my sister came with me to write down the information for me. She knew it would be tough for me to be present in the conversation with the physician and also take notes for later. I filled out what felt like a ten-page document which went through all of your previous health history, and with a chronic illness that could take ages. My fertility doctor was friendly with a way of making you feel comfortable through humour, he respected the fact that I was a nurse and didn't water down any medical terminology, he referred to me as a colleague considering we were both in the medical field which made me feel valued. He talked about absolutely everything that I should know in terms of egg banking, from success rates of eggs vs embryos, sperm donor websites, the cost of egg banking, the stress that eggs banking could put on a person, with my chances of issues increasing because of sickle cells. I left that appointment overwhelmed and so confused. I had so many options but I had no idea which would be best. This is where things got complicated. I could opt to freeze embryos with a random sperm donor and have to explain to my future children that I chose their daddy off of a sperm donor website and they may never meet or know him. Or I could embark on an extremely difficult and awkward conversation, where I ask my boyfriend of two years if I could borrow some sperm. It was a difficult decision to make at 25, unmarried and within a time constraint.

Once home I found my parents peacefully enjoying the warm weather whilst reclining in chairs on our backyard deck. I shared the information from the appointment with my family, and the looks on their face pointed to one thing, almost as if the only thing they heard me say was that egg freezing is especially dangerous for sickle cell patients due to the high level of hormones I would have to take. Hormones can increase your body's risk for blood clots and considering I was frequently having pain crises; it did seem like a bad idea to potentially increase that risk. My parents are protectors, they didn't want to see me going through any more pain and suffering than I was already. They told me they'd think about all of the information I had presented to them and get back to me tomorrow about their thoughts.

Later that evening I went to go and visit my boyfriend, the weather had shifted from a nice warm sunny day to a windy evening with extreme weather warnings. I had my piece of paper from the doctor's visit on my passenger seat as I approached his place. It was so windy that I struggled to open the door. Once I finally opened it up you wouldn't believe what happened, before I even had a chance to get out of the car a gust of wind came into my car, grabbed the lone piece of paper on my passenger seat and swept it out of my car and into the street. I jumped to my feet and began to chase it but the wind was much faster than I could even dream of. I hoped it would get stuck to a tree or behind another car so I would have a chance to get it but no. With my head hanging low I knocked on his door with tears in my eyes. With a concerned look on his face, he asked me what was wrong, I told him what happened and almost instantly took to the street running and searching for my paper. After about ten minutes he returned without the paper, feeling bad that it had been carried away. At the time I felt like that paper had my answer on it and was devastated by it being swept away in such a freakishly unusual way. Now I think of this situation as pretty funny because if anyone was looking out of their front window, they definitely got a live cartoon show. We spent the evening together, discussing options and bouncing ideas off of each other. The thought crossed my mind to dive into that awkward "can I have your sperm" conversation but I figured I'd been through enough emotionally for one day. I decided it would be best to table the conversation until another opportune time.

After over a month of going back and forth in my head, talking to life coaches, counsellors, psychologists and of course God. I finally decided that I was going to go forward with freezing my eggs despite the risk. I just wasn't willing to let my body get irradiated and potentially fry all of my reproductive organs without having a plan B. When you're as crazy type A as I am there is no room for not having a plan B. I figured it was best to simply freeze my eggs on my own, despite the decrease success rates, I decided to trust that God will provide and that things will work out the way God designed them to.

I used to find comfort in the fact that other people I knew had gone through IVF and could provide me with information. There was a part of me that envied other people that have gone through this process with a partner. In the waiting room I felt awkward sitting there alone with a huge decision on my shoulders, while I saw couples holding hands, or a head rested on a shoulder. I didn't realize it was possible to feel alone in a crowded waiting room of people. My fertility doctor referred me to the Calgary clinic in hopes that I could receive some funding, Edmonton didn't have any programs or charities in place to subsidize the cost. Although Calgary was three hours away and it would be such a hassle to go back and forth, I decided that with a $10,000 bill in front of me I was willing to try anything that would help. My physician at the regional fertility clinic in Calgary was great, she made me feel heard and also provided personalized medical advice to me. This initial meeting with her was just to get acquainted and then she provided me with what the next steps would be. Pretty much once I got my period then everything would be a go.

Medications

Medications/Injections I was on:

Acetylsalicylic acid (ASA) - anti-inflammatory properties

Folic Acid - helps prevent birth defects

Gonal F - boost my follicle stimulating hormones

Luveris - boost luteinizing hormone and in turn help my eggs grow and mature

Fragmin - anti coagulation properties

Superfact - stimulate ovaries to make estrogen

Antibiotics - protect me against bacteria exposure during egg retrieval

Valium - good night's sleep the night before retrieval day

Let me walk you through what my egg collection process looked like:

Dates	Medications	Interventions
September 8, 2017		Day 1 of period call clinic
September 9, 2017		Blood test and ultrasound
September 10, 2017	ASA Folic Acid 175IU Gonal F 75IU Luveris Fragmin	

September 11, 2017	ASA Folic Acid 175IU Gonal F 75IU Luveris Fragmin	
September 12, 2017	ASA Folic Acid 175IU Gonal F 75IU Luveris Fragmin	
September 13, 2017	ASA Folic Acid 175IU Gonal F 75IU Luveris Fragmin	
September 14, 2017	ASA Folic Acid 125IU Gonal F 75IU Luveris Fragmin	Blood test and ultra-sound
September 15, 2017	ASA Folic Acid 125IU Gonal F 75IU Luveris Fragmin	

September 16, 2017	ASA Folic Acid 125IU Gonal F 75IU Luveris Fragmin	Blood test and ultra-sound
September 17, 2017	ASA Folic Acid 125IU Gonal F 75IU Luveris Fragmin	Blood test and ultra-sound
September 18, 2017	Superfact Injection #1 1mg @2100 Cetrotide 0.25mg @1300 Antibiotics Fragmin 5,000 IU	Blood test and ultra-sound
September 19, 2017	Fragmin 5,000IU @0800 Superfact injection #2 @0900 1mg Clear fluids from midnight/ sleeping pill	Blood test @ 0700
September 20, 2017	Antibiotics Fragmin 5,000IU 6 hrs post retrieval	Retrieval day @ 0800

I remember looking at the giant bag of medical supplies, not really believing that I was going to be able to inject myself. Yes, I'm a nurse, however I prefer to be on the giving end of the injection and not the receiving. The first time I had to stick myself I prepared the medication, swabbed off my stomach with an alcohol swab, removed the syringe cap, pinched an inch of fat off my stomach and then gave myself a pep talk. It sounded kind of like this. "Okay Revée, this should be easy, you know the technique because you do it all the time at work. You're very pain tolerant, so you can do this. It's as simple as 1, 2, 3." Then I chickened out and didn't actually puncture my skin. Again, I counted myself 1, 2, 3! No dice.

I was shocked, because how could me of all people be nervous about a tiny little needle in my belly fat when I get massive large bore needles into my chest every seven weeks? Once that thought crowded my mind, the nerves wore off and again I counted 1, 2, 3, poked my belly and slowly injected the medication. I was proud that I got through this, unfortunately this one small poke was only a drop in bucket of the almost 40 injections that I gave myself in total during this process. Poking myself was hard, but at times I found the hardest part really to be finding an appropriate time to give myself these injections. They had to be administered between 1PM and 5PM every day and at the same time daily. That doesn't sound too difficult but when you are working an 8AM – 4PM job that's tougher than you think. Although I finished at 4PM, it left me with only an hour to dash out of my office, cross the street to where I parked my car, crawl home in slow moving rush hour traffic, sprint to bathroom and begin preparing my medications.

There were a few days when I had appointments or meetings after work that wouldn't leave me anytime to go home and give myself my injections. I had to do a few injections in the bathroom of the clinic I was working at, it was clean but still a germaphobes nightmare. I'd search the floor for an individual bathroom when I could disinfect and set up shop. I like to keep my work and personal life separate, however in this situation I had to let my manager in on what was going on because the days I was required at the clinic in Calgary were so unpredictable. I was told to expect to be there every one to three days, so that didn't leave an abundance of room for planning your life. I was so fortunate I worked part-time and had a manager that really took the time to understand my situation. As time went on, I began to feel heavy, feel my stomach bloating more and more and of course my chest exploded. Not only did all of these hormones affect my body physically, they also were beginning to affect me emotionally. I'm already a softy, but these hormones surged me into another realm, I was moody, tearful, and couldn't control my emotions. I do have a great poker face when I'm out and about but the moment I came home and could finally breathe I was all over the place. Unfortunately, the person that got the worst of my late-night emotions was my poor boyfriend that would call me every night to see how I was feeling and would have to deal with my sporadic crying or angry rants. I'm thankful that even though I wasn't the easiest person to be around he still wanted to be around.

My Dad

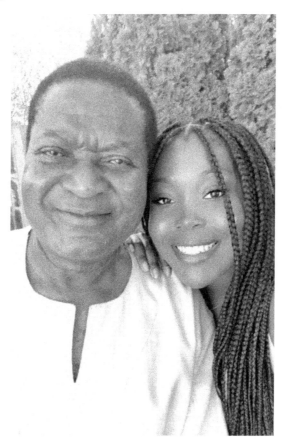

During my fertility treatments, my dad nominated himself to be my personal to and from Calgary chauffeur. My dad is someone who never, I repeat never takes time off so we he does it's a big deal. My mom was out of town and he figured that he'd be able to step up and help me. When we were getting ready to go, we didn't have any idea how many days I'd have to spend there so packing was tough. Our mornings were early and busy. The hotel we stayed at had a delicious continental breakfast that we always took advantage of. The clinic began doing blood work at 7:30AM and ultrasounds between 7:30AM – 9:00AM. Which doesn't sound too bad, but here's the catch, there's no appointment times. You just have to show up and are seen on a first come first serve basis. Here's the second catch, the fertility clinic doors opened at 6:00AM, it was then that you were able to go into the building and take a number. The third catch was, hormonal women who are cranky and just want a baby don't play around. The first day I casually showed up at 7:00AM because it made sense that if it opened at 7:30AM, you'd be 30 minutes early aka the first one? Boy was I wrong, I think that day I was number 30 and trust me it only took that one time to realize how things really worked in the fertility world. From that day on, my dad and I would go at 6:00AM, get a number, go back to our hotel to have breakfast then casually mosey into the clinic around 7:15AM feeling smug that we were ahead of the game. I know I was feeling smug but I don't think my dad cared what number we got as long as I eventually got seen. To my surprise the one day we got there at 6:15AM which is still us being over achievers we were number ten which just blew my mind that everyone was that eager. After a while I began to recognize familiar faces in the waiting room, indicating that these people were probably at the same stage in their fertility journey as I was.

From time to time, I found that my dad and I would get the weirdest stares, I'd comb through my mind wondering what could be so weird about me, for a while it made me feel insecure because people were judging me due to my age. Soon my wondering was answered when a patient that I frequently saw at the clinic leaned over and asked me "so how long have you and your husband wanted children?" I looked at her in complete confusion, wondering what husband? And who says I'm trying to have children now? Then all of a sudden it clicked, the weird looks, and raised eyebrows were because everyone thought that my 65-year-old dad was my husband, which was wrong on so many levels. I laughed for a second before I leaned back over saying "that's my dad, I'm from Edmonton so he's, my chauffeur". The woman looked embarrassed but soon realized that I wasn't offended at all, rather thought it was hilarious. We both had a nice much needed laugh in such a tough time. You'd patiently wait for the nurse to call you name, for your blood work. My name would be called and I felt bad for everyone that came after me because I knew what lay ahead for the poor nurse that wouldn't be able to get my bloodwork. It was always a process, took preheating my arm, the lecture about drinking enough water (which I always did), two-four pokes and then eventually my bloodwork was done in the time it generally takes for three people to get theirs done. After blood work I would go back to the seating area until I was called by the next nurse that would take me into the examination room for my vaginal ultrasound. Yes, these ultrasounds are just as unpleasant as you would imagine, a hard cold wand being inserted into your vagina would be. The pressure was intense as I was already feeling tender since beginning the hormone injections but I didn't have a choice but to be strong and just get through it. Based on the way your follicles were looking and the bloodwork done earlier, this is when you might get a change in medication dosing and be instructed when to come back to the clinic for another examination. To my surprise there came a time when I was asked to come back the next day for 4 days straight, at that point I might as well have moved to Calgary. My dad and I spent our mornings to early afternoons at the clinic, afternoon napping, early evening hitting the mall and late evenings eating and preparing to do it all over again.

Retrieval

I always knew the IVF wasn't easy but I didn't realize how stressful it was. A few nights before the retrieval you are expected to give yourself a superfact injection at exactly 9PM and then again exactly 12 hours from that time which would be at 9AM. So that you had both doses in exactly 24 hrs before your expected retrieval. To my understanding this medication shuts off the production of estrogen and allows your eggs to separate from the follicle. I was paranoid about potentially messing up the times and the medication to working as expected. Thankfully that didn't happen. I woke up the morning of the retrieval day extremely exhausted, feeling extremely bloated to the point of pain and I swear five pounds heavier. To get out of bed I had to roll onto my side, slowly lower my legs off the side of the bed, use my left elbow to push me up while my right hand pulled on the mattress for support. I waddled to the bathroom to get ready, eventually got dressed and waddled out of the hotel room with my dad. When we got to the fertility clinic, we were taken into a back area which looked like an OR prep unit. As per usual it was next to impossible to get and IV in me. After about 4 missed pokes by various RNs, the doctor that would be doing my retrieval had to come in and get it done. I had IV fluids and antibiotics pumped into me and then I was wheeled into the OR and helped up onto the operating table. The nurse places my legs in the highest set of stirrups I've ever seen, which would have been very awkward if I hadn't just spent the last three weeks in this position getting vaginal ultrasounds. But this time was different for me, I was nervous beyond believe and scared. I was given an IV sedative and pain medication. This was my first experience with conscious sedation. For me I don't get why they call it conscious sedation, I wasn't sedated at all, I was wide awake and the fact that the "sedation" wasn't touching me was only adding to my stress. I was told to give it a min and see what happens. The procedure began and I was still wide awake with anxiety rising. As someone who has experienced pain my entire life, I didn't expect an abundance of pain, but oh man I was wrong. I would have to say this was the most sharp and intense pain I have ever experienced, easily a 10/10 on the pain scale. By the end of the procedure, I was given about triple the starting dose. I don't remember much of what happened after the retrieval. All I remember was being extremely nauseated but still begging my dad that we should drive home to Edmonton that day. At point all I wanted to do was just be home in my own bed. The next few days of recovery were tough, I felt very sick and I was told due to the large number of eggs that were collected I was at risk of Ovarian Hyper Stimulation Syndrome (OHSS). Long story short all of those follicles that released eggs, could now fill with fluid causing your ovaries to become very swollen and painful. I ended up getting mild to moderate OHSS, at that point I didn't really care, all that mattered to me is that it was done and I now had a backup plan.

CHAPTER TEN

GETTING READY

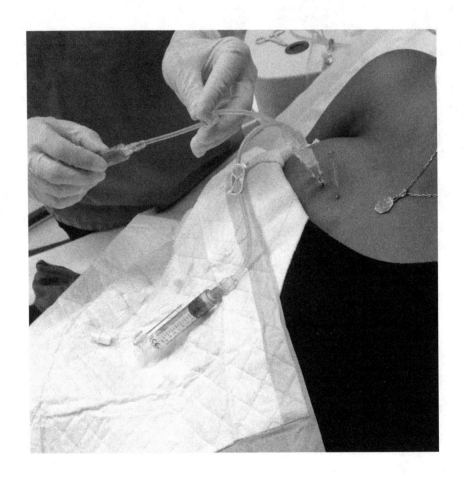

Transplant Workup Phase

The month of October was one of the busiest times I've ever experienced. I stepped away from my nursing job and began my medical leave. I used this month to prepare myself physically for transplant by running errands and buying all of the things that I thought might be helpful during my first 100 days. I spent time with family, my boyfriend and friends because at that point I didn't even know if I was going to make it out of Calgary. I was thrown a beautiful surprise going away party and received a lovely video of all my closest friends sending me well wishes so I could play it when things got tough. My niece and nephew drew me pictures that I could keep at my bedside. I spent lots of time at church, trying to strengthen my relationship with God. The most of my time was spent trying to complete my pre-transplant appointment list. The majority of my time was spent in appointments, the purpose of this "workup phase" was to collect a baseline of overall health status prior to stem cell transplant. Some days I had up to four appointments and sometimes only one.

Here's a sneak peak of my appointment schedule:

Week 1	CT scan
	Ophthalmologist
	Dentist
	PET scan
	ECG
	Echocardiogram
	X-Ray
Week 2	24 hr urine test
	Ophthalmologist
	Psychology
	Massage therapy 2
	A 2-day trip to Calgary that consisted of a tour of unit 57, pharmacy meeting, RN teaching, bloodwork, psychosocial assessment, physician meet up and dietitian

Week 3	Blood work
	Laser eye surgery
	Massage therapy
	Red cell exchange
	Comprehensive phone review with physician

My sister, my mom and I ventured on a two-day trip to Calgary. My sister also had a few appointments she has to attend as my donor. This trip like every other trip there seemed like it provided us with clarity that put us at ease however at the same time the fact that transplant was only weeks away was terrifying. I remember being told to "bulk up" before transplant because most people lose quite a bit of weight during this process. I didn't even need to "bulk up", I was so stressed out by everything that was to come that stress eating alone easily provided an extra pre-transplant cushion. Before I knew it, I was sitting on my bedroom floor packing my bags in preparation for Calgary. I had a bag for clothes and another suitcase for activities. My clothing suitcase pretty much consisted of all of the comfiest outfits I could find. I brought games like monopoly, uno, jenga and cards. I was gifted a plethora of colouring books, pencil crayons, journals and other stationery so I brought all of that.

I packed a separate bag that was going to be my hospital bag. If you are preparing for an extended hospital stay and are not sure what to bring this list might help.

- Slippers - because who wants to walk around in socks or attempt to lace up shoes every time you have to get up

- One comfy outfit - incase I was feeling fancy and wanted to bust out of the standard hospital gown

- A good book to curl up and read when visitors have left for the night

- A reading light that clips onto your book, a good way to avoid turning on the blinding bright lights each room is equip with

- A heated blanket because we all know that the hospital heated blankets lose their heat in ten minutes

- An extension cord because finding a socket that was close enough to my bed and wasn't going to short circuit my medical equipment was tough

- A housecoat to stay warm

- A stack of thoughtful cards I received from supportive friends and family members to boost your mood

- A few inspirational plaques to stay motivated when the going got rough

- Most importantly I packed my bible. From the start I knew that this was going to be a tough journey that would require me to draw strength from God.

Transplant Conditioning Phase

Home Away From Home

In the blink of an eye my bags were packed and I was heading to Calgary to begin this wild stem cell transplant adventure. My family and I arrived at the condo we would be staying at on November 1st, in the afternoon leaving us enough time to get settled and prepare for admission. As nervous as I was for what was to come, I knew God's hand was in the midst of everything. Through a friend I was blessed with meeting the most lovely woman during my workup phase. This woman is the definition of an angel. She selflessly allowed my family and I to stay at one of her condos just off the bow river. Let me backtrack a little bit, it was going to cost $1500 per month for a tiny two-bedroom outdated apartment that was attached to the hospital. Yes, it had its conveniences because you were walking distance from the hospital but paying that much for the almost four months, we'd have to stay there was going to be tough especially because I was going to be on short term disability. Her place was on the top floor of a condo complex that overlooked the bow river, it had a huge bedroom with a bathroom, laundry room, and office just steps away from it. The kitchen was grand and fully stocked, when I say fully stocked this is no exaggeration. The drawers and cupboards were full of cups, plates, utensils, cooking gadgets, pots and pans. The cabinets were full of non-perishable foods and the fridge/freezer both were full of condiments and frozen treats. The living room had a comfy couch with extra sitting chairs, a TV and tons of games, books and magazines. The dining room had a 6-seater table that provided a perfect view of the bow river while also beside the charming fireplace. Just off the living room there were stairs leading up to the loft style bedroom. This room was just as beautiful as the one downstairs but it had an attached bathroom with a double sink, water closet, giant standing shower with gorgeous blue tiles that led up to the vaulted roof lined with numerous skylights. This was about the time when I said pinch me is this place real? I was in awe of how beautiful this place was and felt even more blessed that I had the opportunity to stay somewhere so beautiful while I recovered. There was no time limit on how long we stayed there, we were told that it was ours until we were ready to go. Now that you have a better idea of where we stayed, I'll move on.

Pampering

The night before my admission I was pampered by my family, everyone was waiting on every want and need so naturally I took advantage of it and suggested that we order in Chinese food. I am completely obsessed with Chinese food and I was told that once I start chemo and radiation my immune system will not allow me to eat outside food, so I figured it was now or never. I made the joke at the dinner table after we prayed over the food that this was like the last supper. Everyone laughed at my silliness, but there was a part of me that wasn't joking when I said that, there was a part of me that really was uncertain if I was ever going to leave the hospital after I entered it the next day. We enjoyed our meal, watched some TV and enjoyed each other's company. It was a long day so we opted for an early night knowing we would all have to be up bright and early. That night I couldn't sleep. I was full of thoughts, I was so excited that it was finally here while at the same time so stressed out that it all begins tomorrow, but mostly I was hopeful and optimistic about the potential to be cured. So, I decided to keep my mind positive, my faith high and my eye on the prize.

CHAPTER ELEVEN

ADMISSION DAY

We started admission morning with a family prayer and then headed off to the Tom Baker Cancer Centre. We wandered around the hospital in the most lost fashion of course until we finally found the area we had to be at. Unsure if we were in the right place, I peeked my head around the corner of an office door and said Hi. Just as I did that, I was greeted by two very friendly nurses with giant smiles on their faces. They took me into a small room that had a stretcher, a sterile field and some medical equipment. I don't know why but laying there on that bed while the nurses assessed my vessels to figure out which one would be best to insert the peripherally inserted central catheter (PICC) line into made me feel nervous. You'd think because of my lifetime of being poked and prodded that a simple procedure wouldn't even phase me, wrong I was so nervous that I was given Ativan to help with the anxiety. For anyone that doesn't know what a PICC line is, it is a long catheter that is placed in a vein usually in your arm that extends all the way to the inferior vena cava which is the large vessel that carries blood to your heart. This provides your care team with central access for medications, fluids and blood products. Once the line was in and secured, I was on my way. I looked over at my left arm that felt heavy and was covered in gauze, tape, and a new gadget that would be with me for my time in Calgary. Step one was now complete, step two consisted of heading to my new home on unit 57 and being admitted. We got off the elevators and stood in a circle outside of unit 57. I looked up at the unit doors and there was a big sign that said "no children allowed on the unit." I mean I understand that children can be a breeding ground for bacteria, but they really couldn't come and visit me. I wondered if this was the last time, I'd see my niece and nephew for 100 days or maybe ever the last time I'd ever see them again.

At the time myself or my family members had any idea what was ahead of us. We were extremely hopeful that after all of this I would have the chance to live a sickle cell free life. A real life, one that didn't consist of around the clock hospital admissions, exams and appointments. A life where I didn't have to be afraid of everything and constantly live in a state of high alert. This thought, this hope, and this faith in God is what we had to hold onto to keep us going.

P.S I Love You

I looked around at the faces that surrounded me, there was my mom, my dad, my sister, my brother-in-law, my boyfriend, my niece and my nephew. Seeing them all try to fight back tears and hide the worry they really felt while my dad led us in prayer was tough. Before we headed inside, I dug inside my travel bag and pulled out five letters. Each envelope was addressed to a family member. They all looked at me shocked and confused what I was handing them. Although I was faithful, I looked at both sides of the coin. One side said that everything was going to go well and I'd be the happiest and healthiest I've ever been at the end of this. The other side of the coin, the side that I tried to suppress and ignore was the ugly truth that God's plan for my life could be death while searching for a cure. It was a scary thought that I definitely tried to avoid but the small chance that I could reject my sisters stem cells, end up with graft vs host disease, or run into a post-transplant infection that had the potential to kill me was terrifying.

To combat that fear I decided to be as prepared as I possibly could, I wrote letters to all of my immediate family members and my boyfriend telling them just how much I loved and cared for them. It's sad to think of it now, I truly believed that those letters were going to be a keepsake for my family if anything bad happened to me. Unfortunately, my brother couldn't get off work to make it for my admission day so he got his letter at a later date.

While everyone was reading their letters, I gave my niece and nephew a letter as well and a pack of stickers. At the time Gabrielle was five and Malakai just turned two so I read them their letter but obviously the most important thing for them was playing with the pack of stickers. I gave them both a long loving hug and a kiss, as I released Gabrielle from my arms and she continued to hold tight my eyes started to fill with tears. It was this moment I realized that Gabriele knew she might not see her auntie for a while. I thought to myself, that hug was necessary for me to remember why I need to fight for health and for a better life.

"I gave my auntie the longest hug ever because I didn't know when we'd play together again" - Gabrielle (Niece).

That hug reminded me that I was deeply loved and there was someone out there that needed me. Although short and over analyzed, that moment is where I got my fight, drive and motivation to get through this from. For anyone that is reading this and are in the midst of a tough time or about to embark on a journey whether it is health related or not, remember we all have something to fight for. We all have a reason to keep on pushing forward, whether that reason is a family member, friend, child, job or responsibility. I urge you to find your reason and trust me you can overcome anything. Maybe take a moment to write down your reason. Write down your why and let's hold on tight.

"Watching Revée walk through the doors of unit 57 made me realize that as much as we all are behind her, she was the only one that had to physically endure what was to come next. Even though we all acted confident, none of us knew what the outcome was. So, we handed her life to God and prayed for the best" - Eddy (Brother-in-law).

Capturing The Moment

Then I took a deep breath and I walked through those doors. Waiting for me in my room was the Alberta Health Services (AHS) camera crew, they were tasked with the job of capturing important moments during my journey. The crew consisted of two men, one would be the interviewer and the other was the videographer/photographer. Before anything got started, I sat down on my bed with cameras pointed at me and began answering interview questions. My mom, dad, sister and boyfriend all stood along the entryway of the room and watched intently. I was asked to share a bit of back story, and a few questions about what was planned for the day. After we finished, my nurse for the day came in and began my admission. She put my admission band on and then I realized this is it, I can no longer run for the hills. I've had many ID bracelets in my lifetime but this one felt different, this one felt more permanent.

Chemotherapy

After my head-to-toe assessment was completed, blood drawn and medications administered, I knew there was only one thing left to do. Chemotherapy or immunosuppressive agent, I've heard Alemtuzemab referred to as both. Whatever it was, chemo or immunosuppression, I knew that it was going to do damage to my body. I was nervous and my nurse knew that, she reassured me that it was going to be a "little pinch" and shouldn't be too painful than any other subcutaneous injection. Trust me I wasn't afraid of a little subcut needle, little did she know I just finished weeks of self-injections for my fertility treatments. I was afraid of the effects and the power that little syringe packed. She reassured me that I was going to be given two test doses, which were only a fraction of the real dose they intended to give me. Pretty much the dose I was getting was just for my body to get adjusted to the medication. That was the type of reassurance I needed. I took my pre- medications which consisted of Hydrocortisone which decreases your body's immune system response, Diphenhydramine to manage symptoms like hives, rash, itchiness, running nose or watery eyes, Tylenol, Ondansetron to control the nausea and Ranitidine to decrease stomach acid. Then my regular morning meds were Potassium, Folic acid to support red blood cell production, and Valacyclovir an antiviral. I laid down on my bed, my nurse pinched an inch of my stomach fat and then slowly injected the medication. This was the first step and I just took it. I braced myself for what I thought was the beginning of the end. I braced myself for what I saw in all of the movies that depicts what happens to you during chemo. Ultimately, I braced myself for the nausea, vomiting and weakness but it didn't come. Partially because I expected it to be instant and partially because I expected it to be cinematic. The day went by and I sat on the window cill of my hospital room that overlooked a portion of the hospital. My boyfriend and I sat there and people watched while we passed the time. We smiled back at each other and made jokes but in the back of our minds we knew our relationship was about to get real. It wasn't going to be about fancy dates, cute pictures and outings for a while.

Night Pass

The first day went by much faster than I expected, all of a sudden it was 6PM and my physician came into my room and told me that because I was doing so well, I could go home for the night. I was so excited because when I walked in to the unit, I didn't think I was going to be able to leave for at least another 30 days if ever. My family was a little worried about me going back to the condo with the kids being around since if I was on the unit there was to be no contact with children. My dad especially was hesitant, or resistant to me going home for the night, he questioned the doctors carefully getting him to outline the pros and cons of me going home vs staying. At the time I was irritated because I just wanted to be around my family but now, I do see that he just wanted to keep me safe. The doctor said that patients actually heal a lot faster when they are in and out of the hospital because being in the hospital makes people believe that they are ill. In some cases, you do need hospital attention and it's not safe to leave, however in my experience I do feel that the longer I have been in the hospital the longer it takes me to bounce back. Laying in a bed all day, wearing a hospital gown, and being confined to a tiny room sounded much less appealing than spending time with family in a gorgeous condo with a view. So, after much debate my dad was convinced that it was a good idea and I grabbed my overnight bag and headed home.

When we got home, I sat on the couch wrapped in a warm blanket, I soon noticed that my whole family was in the living room but no one wanted to sit too close to me. Everyone was extra cautious as if my immune system was already at zero and they were going to infect me. We were never really sure how sick I was going to get or how things were going to go so we keep a close watch on everything that could be a potential issue. Around 9PM, I began feeling cold and had the chills. The physician said that this might happen but it wasn't anything to be alarmed about unless I developed a fever with it. So, for the time been I ignored it because I so badly did not want to go back to the hospital. I wanted to prove to my hesitant parents that I was much stronger than they thought. Unfortunately, that didn't happen, not long after the chills began, I developed a fever that forced me back to the hospital. I was scared that night because the physician had just said to look out for those side effects but I didn't know if that meant I was having a negative reaction or if this was bound to happen to everyone. I was reassured upon arrival that what I was experiencing was just my body getting used to the Alemtuzemab. Now I was back in my hospital bed by midnight, looking up at the roof thinking that I was already shook up and this was only the beginning. This was day one of my seven-days conditioning phase, this was all about preparing my body for the transplant. I thought to myself if this is just the prep what will the rest be like?

What Next?

My next few days looked very similar. They started with 5AM blood work by the phlebotomist that loved flicking all of the bright lights on the moment he walked into my room. Then on to the nurse's assessment which I was always half asleep for after the abrupt awakening by the phlebotomist. I would be checked from head to toe, and asked questions while barely understanding them out of exhaustion. Next step was breakfast, we all know that hospital breakfasts are not the greatest or considered breakfast for champs, however at the Tom Baker Cancer Centre the breakfasts were always amazing to encourage patients to eat. This was the first time I actually looked forward to hospital breakfast. After that comes morning medications and pre-chemo medications. Pretty much once I took these I was out for the afternoon, they put me to sleep almost immediately. The nurse would come in shortly after I took my pre-meds and begin the chemotherapy prep. This process consisted of the nurse donning a gown, gloves, mask and eye shield then preparing the medication. I would watch her and wonder how she had protected herself from head to toe from this medication but that same medication was about to be injected into me. I always got a cold pack prior to injection because it burned as she injected it and the cold would take the edge off. Once that was over, I usually spent the rest of my morning sleeping and then woke up for lunch. After lunch was always different, some days I was able to go home for the afternoon but expected to return by the evening or would leave in the evening and stay at the condo overnight. The first few days of chemotherapy went by and all I would experience was chills, night sweats and fever. All of the side effects that people talk about experiencing was no match for me. I felt invincible, I felt superhuman, I felt bionic. This is where my nickname "bionics" was born. It was during the first week of treatment that my family started calling me bionics because they were just as shocked as I was that I wasn't feeling any of the expected signs of chemotherapy. Every evening that I would get a pass I would ask someone to go on a walk with me along the bow river. I would be able to keep top stride and pace with my family members and dance around with my niece and nephews. This gave me confidence that whatever was ahead of me I would be able to withstand because I was stronger than I thought. A few days later my bionic confidence bubble was popped by total body irradiation. Total body irradiation (TBI) is a treatment that uses high powered rays to destroy cells. It affects the targeted (abnormal or bad) cells as well as your normal cells, similarly to chemotherapy. People often get radiation to a localized area, however in my case I was receiving total body irradiation, so from head to toe.

CHAPTER TWELVE

TOTAL BODY IRRADIATION

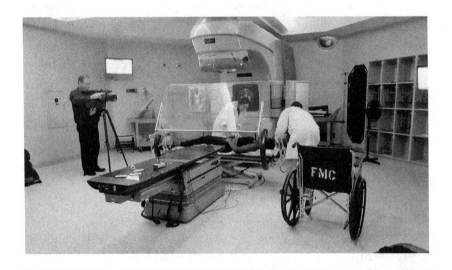

"Radiation was the last day of Revée's conditioning but it seemed to be one of the more nerve-wracking days for all of us. This was such uncharted territory. We wondered if she would get burnt? What if her eggs don't survive? Is it possible the radiation could do more damage than intended?" - Eddy (Brother-in-law)

I woke up that morning feeling very hopeful knowing that this was going to be the last piece of my conditioning phase, then I would be granted a rest day before transplant. The idea that I had already survived five days of chemo and was feeling just fine made me think that radiation wasn't going to be any different. That morning, mom, dad, sister, brother-in-law, niece, nephew and I gathered around the kitchen island and bowed our heads in prayer. We headed to the hospital blasting gospel praise and worship music while singing at the top of our lungs. We started this tradition as we drove to Calgary and wanted to put God in the center of this experience so I felt it was necessary every morning to remind myself and those around me that God has a plan. When we got to the hospital, I went back upstairs to my room for my morning assessment and then immediately it was off to the ground floor in the radiation oncology department. We waited by the giant glass windows that overlooked a hill and the bow river in the distance. I looked around and saw so many different people also waiting for their names to be called, some were in wheelchairs, some sleeping in recliners, some bundled in blankets and some watching TV. I wondered what all of their stories were, I wondered the type of cancers they had, if it was their first time around or if they've done this before.

All of sudden I heard a man call my name, I remembered him from the video conference we had over the summer where I pretty much grilled him on everything radiation. I stood up and followed him, with my entourage behind me. He showed us all of the computer equipment and how they control the radiation machine from there. It was fascinating to see and understand the other side of radiation but the unfortunate part for me was that I was going to be the person on the receiving end. Then he walked us all into a room with a black stretcher in the middle of it with a glass covering. I saw the giant radiation machine that was almost to the roof and wider than a 100-year-old oak tree. This is when the fear set in and I realized what I was about to do. I was given the opportunity to go to the bathroom before the treatment started because it would take about two hours to set up and take down. I remember running to the bathroom in panic, I felt dizzy and I could feel the cold sweat dripping down my body.

"I was pleased by the level of care and compassion that the radiation technologists demonstrated. They knew that we all were nervous about this procedure and took the time to walk us through how total body irradiation worked. They allowed the entire family into the control room (even though there were 6 of us) to understand and observe what Revée was about to go through. This made our entire family feel slightly more at ease. We weren't the ones who were about to get irradiated and we were this stressed. Imagine how Revée was feeling. Just before the procedure I caught Revée in the hallway. Even though she had a smile on her face you could see the fear in her eyes. I gave her a hug and said "Relax Revée, it's going to be okay," I hoped my hug was enough to send her off knowing we were all behind her." - Eddy (Brother-in-law).

I returned back to the radiation suite feeling just as nervous as I was before but with the confidence that everything was going to be alright. My sister laughed at me because she claims that even though I thought I was smiling it was the fakest most terrified smile she'd ever seen on me but was still proud that I forced one out. The AHS camera crew was waiting for me in the room so they could get some footage of my radiation set up. I laid on my back as the technologists positioned and repositioned, strapped me down, packed weighed bags around me and then finally covered me with a glass shield. The moment that glass came down I knew it was game time. I was instructed not to move a muscle to ensure that the dose was delivered evenly to each area of my body. The thought of not being able to move added more stress to the situation. In the overhead microphone I heard the technicians talk to me, "remember we can see and hear you so if you need anything just shout." I said OKAY back to them and then another voice said "okay ready for take-off" with much hesitation I said as ready as I'll ever be.

Music

I was allowed to hook my phone up to their sound system so I opted for my praise and worship playlist. Almost simultaneously my music started playing and the machine started humming, closed my eyes and prayed. I could feel my eyes swell up with tears but I forced myself to stay focused on the music and the lyrics. I had hoped that I would fall asleep but unfortunately high stress Revée wouldn't allow that to happen. I remember watching the way the machine swung and hovered over me back and forth, but after watching for a while I started to think of the damage the radiation was doing to me. I watched the green laser go over my body and when it got to my face, I'd squeeze my eyes shut and it would turn my eyelids purple. After the first few times I realized I just had to accept it, I couldn't escape it, I just had to lay here and hope that the damage wouldn't be too bad. After about 45 minutes the technicians came in, released me from my bondage, but only to flip me on to my stomach so my back side could get irradiated. It was the same as before, I was positioned, repositioned, strapped down and then packed with weights. Now my head sat in a little donut pillow and I had the view of the century - the floor. Honestly the floor view was better than getting to watch the show because watching the show gave your mind time to wander but with the floor there was nothing to be seen. Although I was bored and tired, I still wasn't able to sleep, so I sang along to my music and exercised my patience.

Side Effects

For the last time the technicians came into the room to release me and this time no more positions, I was done. They helped me sit up and I could feel the room spinning around me. I couldn't get up without assistance and my legs felt like they were going to crumble under my weight. I was put in a wheelchair because I felt absolutely exhausted and I was beginning to feel a headache developing, as well as the onset of nausea. Unfortunately for me my PICC line had been hurting really badly and had a huge bump around it so I was been sent straight to ultrasound so they could get a better look at whatever was going on. My mom came with me so I didn't have to be alone and helped me up onto the table. As the ultrasounds progressed, I could feel the slight headache becoming more of a pounding headache that you couldn't ignore. By the time I was back upstairs in my hospital room I felt horrible, my headache became unbearable, it was light and sound sensitive, my weakness was so bad that I had to use my IV pole to keep myself sturdy and my nausea became vomiting. I was so sick. This is when reality set in and I didn't feel "bionic" anymore.

That evening I laid in a dark hospital room, in complete silence with my family also in silence at my bedside. My physician came in to see me and I explained to her what I was experiencing. I told her that I've never in my life had a headache quite this bad and her response was "oh that's cause your brain is swollen" we all waited for a second before we responded because we truly were not sure if she was being serious or joking. But she was serious, it was a fact, radiation has made my brain swell which was causing this headache. The realities of just how scary transplant can be was just beginning to set in, I told my family to go home and get some food and rest because if I didn't, they wouldn't. For the rest of the evening they did shifts, which made it that someone would always be around just in case something happened. I did convince them to at least go home to sleep so they would be rested for tomorrow. I spent that night back and forth from the bathroom throwing up and asking God to give me the strength to manage whatever side effects were around the corner.

Rest Day

The next morning, I woke up with the same pounding headache. I was convinced it was never going to go away. I was convinced that the TBI changed my life for the worse. I was convinced that I took the first steps of the longest journey and there was no turning back now. After surviving the first night post radiation I was fortunate enough to have a pass again for my rest day. Rest day is essentially the day before transplant where you don't have any treatments. My wonderful niece and nephew laid beside me in my bed as I complained that my head was hurting and my eyes were closed to avoid the light. My niece offered to get me breakfast or at least something to drink and my nephew rubbed my back. Talk about service! Having them around was a reminder that I needed to get through this because there were these little humans that loved and cared for me. I spent that "rest day" relaxing on the couch and enjoying the gorgeous views that the bow river had to offer. In the evening when I was supposed to be saving my energy, my niece and nephew suggested we dance. Our favourite dance together is cha cha slide. So, in normal 'Auntie Reva' and kids fashion we decided there was no better way to prepare my body and mind for transplant other than dance the cha cha slide. We danced, we laughed and we made a memory that I will never forget. Dancing literally shook my nervousness off and let my anxieties roll right off my shoulders, it was almost like the kids knew auntie needed to chill out.

CHAPTER THIRTEEN

STEM CELL DONATION

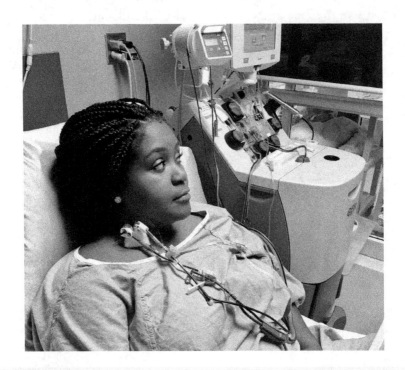

"Being a donor, I felt a significant amount of nervousness and anxiety surrounding my collection. I found myself frequently wondering what if I don't produce enough cells and they have already knocked out my sisters' cells? Then she would be left with no immune system and it would be my fault. Since I was the one who spearheaded all of this, I felt an additional weight on my shoulders, that this process needed to go well or my parents would kill me!" - Stephanie (Sister).

The week leading up to transplant was full of tears, fear and anticipation. While my body was getting prepped for transplant, my sister's body was also getting prepped for her stem cell collection. This was the most important piece of the puzzle. No stem cells would mean no transplant. Stephanie was put on a medication called Neupogen which is a granulocyte colony stimulating factor (GCSF). So, in other words this medication was going to stimulate her bone marrow to produce more stem cells and then release them into the bloodstream. This was to begin via injection so just as I was getting injections so was, she, the only difference was her husband stepped up to the plate to give them to her daily for the five days she had to take it. The first day my sister felt fine after the injections and then the bone pain, weakness and generalized feeling of being unwell increased day by day. It went from a discomfort to a soreness to a bit of pain to her being confined to laying on the couch. I felt bad that she was doing something so selfless for me that was causing her pain. On the last day before her stem cell collection, I remember her asking me if this is what sickle cell pain felt like, I didn't exactly know what she felt but that deep bone pain sounded very familiar. I told her that what she was feeling might only be a fraction of what sickle cell pain felt like. Us just talking about sickle cell pain reminded me that I was putting myself through all of this because I never wanted to feel that type of pain again.

"The GCSF injections weren't too bad. I recruited my husband
to help me with the injections because injecting yourself isn't
easy. So, nurse Eddy to the rescue made them painless and easy.
Initially I didn't feel any "different' and I wondered if it was even
working. As the days went on and I continued with the injections
I began to experience low back pain, hip pain. It progressed into
an overall fatigue and heaviness. My bones felt like they were
under pressure. It wasn't the kind of pain that I have experienced
in the past, this was different, it was bone pain and felt like it was
hurting from the inside out. This the first time I felt like I could
relate to the pain Revée has been experiencing"
- Stephanie (Sister).

My sister provided these tips for potential donors. These are tips that she feels would be helpful to anyone hoping to donate stem cells.

- If you have family talk to them and explain to your family what you being a donor really looks like and how it may impact their family life (i.e., childcare needs, decreased wages due to time off work).

- Talk to your family about the reasons why you think stem cell donation is important, let them understand why you feel the need to do it and discuss what your family's fears might be. Note - Some cultures may have difficulties understanding the stem cell transplant process. My family is originally from Ghana and there are so many misconceptions and myths surrounding the blood collection/donation process. So, you may have to take some extra time to ensure they understand.

- It is important to plan ahead. Knowing that transplant is a full family event and it will affect you mentally as the donor. Ensure that you have a support person other than the recipient where you can share your fears or worries about the process with (i.e., a counsellor, friend or spouse).

- If you have any worries, seek out information from reputable sources. (i.e., watch videos of how the apheresis process works so you have a better understanding. Read about GCSF injections and how it works) If you have concerns don't feel shy to ask your doctor for more information.

- Be prepared for every hospital appointment. Have your questions written out for when you meet with the doctor. It's easy to blank/freeze or get off track when we get to the doctor's appointment.

- Lastly, be thankful that God gave you the opportunity to give life!

CHAPTER FOURTEEN

TRANSPLANT DAY – DAY 0

"All of a sudden the long-awaited day of the stem cell transplant was finally here. I spent the night before endlessly praying to the Almighty Lord to guide the doctors and nurses whom the life of my daughter laid in" – Dad.

I woke up in the morning feeling like I was in a movie and it was D-day. You know that feeling when you've been talking about something and waiting for it to happen for so long and then all of a sudden in the blink of an eye it's right in front of you and you have no idea what to do with it. Well, that was me the morning of transplant. Transplant had been this idea, this far-fetched dream that I had but knew it would never come to fruition. Having a match, moving to Calgary, going through chemo and radiation was all for this day. Everything I've done and experienced in my life has led me to this precise moment. So, all that was left for me was to get out of bed, get dressed and get ready for my world to change. At the time I had no idea how my world was going to change, but I just knew it was going to change. It could be for the better but at the same time it could end up drastically worse. My brother-in-law had a pastor that prayed with us all the way from Ghana, West Africa and my sister also added that on Sunday one of her good friends added my name to a prayer list so there were lots of people praying for me. My current Pastor who barely knew me at the time took the time to pray with myself and my family over the phone. I was overwhelmed with the amount of support I was receiving from so many places that I didn't even expect.

My family and I worshipped God knowing that He got us this far and were faithfully believing that He would continue to keep me throughout the rest of this journey. Once we got to my hospital room, I took a moment with my family to record these last few moments of my old life before transplant. At the time, I thought I was recording it so that I had a memory to watch back later but I realized that subconsciously I was making footage that my family could watch back if I didn't make it out of this. It's crazy how one moment can change the trajectory of your life and oftentimes we have no idea if that will be for our benefit or not. The Alberta Health Services communications team came again to get some footage of this special day. We had another small interview and then it was time.

"As we waited for the transplant to begin the room was quiet and solemn. Despite all of the risks and potential complications that could occur there was no turning back. Seeing my daughter's eyes wide open and excited for the transplant coupled with her beautiful smile made me realize even if I wasn't ready for her to get a transplant, she was" – Dad.

I sat up in the bed covered with my heated blanket. I watched as the nurse created her sterile field, prepared her work space, clipped and twisted lines and pushed pre-medications. It was weird seeing someone else doing what would be my job and I just had to sit there as a patient. My doctor came in and she gave me an update on my blood counts because she knew how much I looked forward to documenting my numbers daily. I looked to my left and the nurse was removing the bag of stem cells from the cooler. She handed me the bag and said "these are your sister stem cells, do you want to take a picture?" I excitedly called my sister out of her seat and we captured a few pictures with this beautiful bag of stem cells. I held this cold bag of gold in my hands and thanked God. It didn't make sense. This little bag was about to change things FOREVER.

Tears of Joy

I handed it back to the nurse, the final checks were completed, she spiked the bag and hung it. I watched the IV tube intently as the clear IV flush became a light reddish brown, and the stem cells got closer and closer to my PICC line site. In that moment I had absolutely no control, my eyes began to swell up and tears rolled down my cheek. At the moment it was a tear of joy. A tear that quickly turned into me sobbing uncontrollably out of happiness and realizing that it was really happening. That a moment that I never ever imagined was happening. I kept repeating "I can't believe this is happening" and "I'm so happy." My sister quickly jumped to her feet and held me tight. All I could say to her was "thank you." My dad then came closer and said "Revée be strong" and asked that we all join him in prayer.

My dad began *"Our Father in Heaven, we thank You so much for making this day possible. We never thought it would happen, but since we had trust in you, since you've been our guardian and since you've guided us through this process, you have taken control of every single procedure. I know the recovery will be as smooth as the preparation to get to this day. Our Lord help these two ladies to be as close to you as possible. Amen."*

I cried through the entire prayer because sitting there hooked up to these stem cells, I could feel the love of God like never before. One of the first prayers I've ever prayed was asking God to cure me of this horrible disease. I was crying out to God and wondering what I did to deserve such a curse. It was praying that the doctors would stop telling me that my organs are becoming more and more affected. In that moment all of these prayers rushed into my mind and I realized they were being answered.

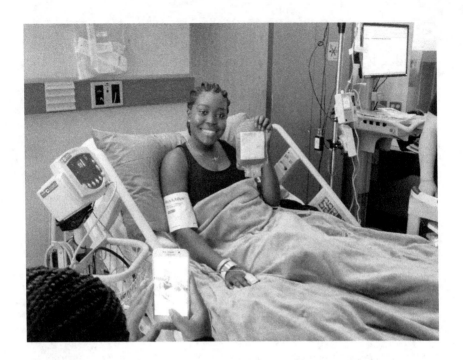

1.5 Hours

In reality transplant is merely an hour and a half infusion and then just like that you had a transplant. That hour and half felt like a lifetime though. I laid there and watched my nurse buzz around, frequently checking vitals, monitoring the infusion and constantly checking my status for transfusion reactions. I had a slight metallic taste in my mouth that I couldn't shake. I told my nurse and she mentioned that a lot of people experience that during their stem cell infusion. She pulled a candy out of her pocket and gave it to me. I am glad she was prepared because I sure wasn't. My infusion seemed pretty straight forward, until it wasn't. I went from convers-ing with my family, laughing and singing to chills. I began to feel a bit cold so I asked for my nurse to plug in my heater blanket. I started it on low, increased to medium and then eventually was on high and still feeling cold. I began shivering and shaking un-controllably, my teeth started chattering despite the extra blankets my nurse was putting on top of my heated one. This is when the fear and panic of transplant began to set in. I could see it on the expressions of my loved ones' faces. They were scared because my carefree straight forward transplant wasn't so straight forward. Additionally, nurses began to enter my room as well as my doctor and then I knew it was serious. I laid in my bed with my mind racing and truly wondering what was going to happen next. I watched my nurse push a few medications into my IV with no effect and then eventually one worked. The chatter of my teeth subsided and my body stopped shaking. I was still cold but I could handle it. The nurse explained to my family that I was experiencing a transfusion reaction called rigors. You'd think as a nurse I'd know exactly what was going on but my nurse brain was left at the entrance of the Tom Baker Cancer Centre. It's funny how things make so much sense in a textbook but when it's happening to you, it doesn't.

After the transplant transfusion completed my whole family and I cheered with excitement and disbelief that it actually happened already. After the transplant I was exhausted, very weak and that terrible post radiation headache began to return. It was a piercing headache that was light and sound sensitive. They tried Tylenol with no effect, Morphine tablets with no effect and eventually what ended up working was IV Morphine. Isn't that insane? I never imagined I'd have a headache bad enough that would require IV narcotics to control it. I was used to IV narcotics for sickle cell crises but definitely not headaches. I was feeling so worn out my family left me to rest that afternoon. To be honest I don't remember much of what the rest of that day consisted of. All I remember was my family taking shifts to come and visit me throughout the day and the night. I just laid in bed feeling horrible and wondering if this was the beginning of the end.

CHAPTER FIFTEEN

ACUTE POST-TRANSPLANT PHASE

Section A: Physical Symptoms

I woke up in the hospital still in disbelief that I had a transplant. I felt a bit off, weak and unstable so I spent the morning lying in bed on the computer. The lab tech came in and drew my blood work, the nurse did her regular head to toe assessment and vital signs check, then eventually the doctors came to check in and see how the first night went. Since things looked good, I got the "okay" for a day pass or overnight pass. I opted for a day pass. It was always nice to go home and enjoy a meal with family. I was still in shock that now as my immune system has just been knocked out, I was still able to go home. But the doctors urged me to spend as much time as possible out of the hospital during this recovery period. So that's what I did. Through the first weeks first transplant I slept at the condo and then went back to the hospital every morning for my daily checks. I was feeling so well since conditioning that I really didn't expect this, it hit me like a ton of red bricks. These ominous effects of transplant that my doctors continually warned me about but I thought I was immune to showed up. My doctors would frequently say enjoy the "good days" because the "bad days" were coming. I guess these were the bad days. It started with headache, weakness, nausea and vomiting, followed by stomach pain and diarrhea, then came the mouth sores, sore throat, taste changes and lack of appetite. Oh, but don't get ahead of yourself, we're not done.

Next was the deep throbbing bone pain aka engraftment, it was shortly followed by skin rashes/ peeling, rectal tearing, scalp pain and last but not least hair loss. I know that's a lot of side effects, so let's break this down. I'll go through each symptom I experienced and how I attempted to combat them. I am no health guru and I am sure there are ways that are better than mine but hopefully this can serve as some helpful tips for anything going through something similar.

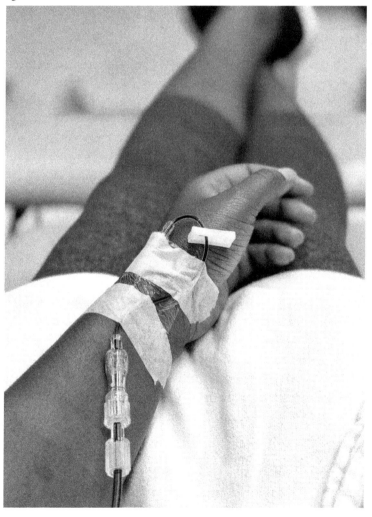

Headache

The headaches weren't those regular ones that you could sleep off, they were prolonged and piercing. No amount of Tylenol or Advil seemed to be enough. Can you imagine that at times the only thing that could control my headaches were narcotics? Yes, people I said narcotics like Morphine and Dilaudid. If I didn't take those then I would feel a constant painful humming headache all day every day. Then again what did I expect? Remember, my brain is swollen from radiation. Really how I managed this was medication almost around the clock, drinking lots of water, decreasing screen time and sometimes just lying-in silence in a dark room.

Weakness & Fatigue

We've all been exhausted, wore out, or muscle fatigued before and felt like we couldn't even take one more step. Well, that was kind of my daily experience. Bending over to tie my shoes or pull up my boots would leave me winded and needing a break. Everyday my mom and I parked and walked through the hospital to my Bone Marrow Transplant Clinic (BMT clinic). A walk that previously took five minutes would now take ten minutes because I would frequently need to stop and take a breather. Sitting up in bed and walking to the bathroom became a tiring event. Imagine going out and having to actually sit on a public toilet, for all of you germa-phobes you understand that you hover over the toilet or you don't use it at all. I was too weak for the hover; I know it was traumatic.

The best advice I can give to fight back fatigue is to be kind to yourself and allow your body the rest it requires. Understand that this is a temporary symptom. Remember temporary is different for everyone. I won't lie, my fatigue took a very long time to shake, it got better as I got stronger but it lingered for one year. You have to find the balance between pushing yourself to be active and rest, but you're smart with a little trial and error and you'll get it!

Pericarditis

This one is not something that post-transplant patients typically experience, however some of us appear to be accident prone. So, what is pericarditis? Well, your heart is held in a sac called the pericardium, so pericarditis is when there is an inflammation of that sac. That causes pain when the heart beats within it. You're probably wondering what, that has to do with transplant and how I was lucky enough to get it. Trust me I am wondering the same thing. Well, it began with intermittent sharp piercing chest pain, that radiated to my shoulder, heart palpitations, and shortness of breath. It took a few trips to the transplant team until we were finally able to crack this code, thankfully it was found after a couple diagnostic tests. I was immediately started on a medication called Colchicine which was to reduce the swelling around the heart. I was really pressed as to how I ended up with this. My transplant team told me that it was likely that I caught a cold from someone who came to visit and was asymptomatic. Somehow the infection that I didn't even know I had traveled from my nose, down my throat and made its way to my heart to infect it. RIGHT! Being immunocompromised does crazy things to you. Now I can make light about this but I was really worried at the time. My transplant team cautioned me that if too much fluid fills this sac, my heart could have trouble beating and we all know what that means. I felt like I was a ticking time bomb or something. Thankfully with a few months of anti-inflammatory medication the pain eventually subsided and I was back to normal!

Section B: Gastrointestinal Changes

Nausea & Vomiting

The nausea was the worst part for me. We've all eaten something bad and became nauseous before. But this was different, it was nausea day in and day out. I was taking Gravol and Zofran (both anti-emetic) every other hour alternating. Even with that I still felt horrible. It was the type of nausea that even after you threw up you still felt sick. It was horrible and I spent most of my days laying on the couch complaining about it.

My advice to cope with this is to have as much bread, crackers and ginger ale as you can. This is your excuse to enjoy carbs guilt free! Electrolyte drinks to help you replace some of the electrolytes you are losing with all the vomiting. I bought an anti-nausea wrist band that is supposed to use pressure points to help manage nausea, to be honest some days I think it worked and others it was no help.

Stomach Pain & Diarrhea

Stomach pain is never fun. It felt like someone had punched me in the stomach. It felt unsettled constantly but eventually I just became used to that uncomfortable feeling. The stomach pain I was told was as a result of the cocktail of medications I was taking as well as my stomach lining shedding. Sounds lovely, doesn't it? What I didn't get used to and never will get used to is the diarrhea. Just as I mentioned that my gastric lining was shedding, everything had to come out somehow. I didn't have normal bowel movement for weeks. Trust me after a while, things begin to get very sore and tender.

There wasn't much I could do for my stomach pain other than placing a heat pad on my stomach, I didn't take any Advil or Tylenol for it because I didn't want to introduce any additional medication into my system since I was already taking enough for an entire family. The transplant team reassured me that this wouldn't last forever but it will take time for my body to settle out. All I can recommend for diarrhea is avoiding hot and spicy foods and of course flushable wipes are a must!

Mouth Sores & Sore Throat

We've all had a canker sore, bit our lip/cheek or burnt our tongue. Essentially the mouth sores you get post-transplant are like having all three of those covering your entire mouth. It sounds super dramatic but I'm telling you it's painful. These sores actually started with the throat for me. At first it was just uncomfortable to swallow food, then started feeling weird to drink water, then eventually it was so painful to swallow. This was half of the reason why eating used to be my favourite quickly became my least favourite activity of the day.

To manage these, I suggest a club soda rinse after every meal to clean out any bacteria, as well as drinking water whenever you can because a painful mouth sucks but a painful mouth that is also dry is worse. If that doesn't work a few other washes worked for me, "pink lady" which is essentially this numbing pink liquid that you swish and spit, it leaves your mouth nice and numb afterwards. Often when I just needed a spot treatment, I would dip a Q-tip into the liquid and rub it on the specific sore areas. But I would have to say that the best of the best is Dr. Akabutu's mouthwash! It's a combination of cooling, numbing and disinfecting all at once. It gave me the most relief ever, I felt like it was God sent. It worked wonders for me so I hope it will do the same for you. If all else fails go back to the basics ice cream, cold smoothies and popsicles are helpful.

Taste Changes & Decreased Appetite

Taste changes was a case of you never knowing how good you have something until you lose it. As a self-proclaimed foodie, not being able to taste the food left me with absolutely no reason to eat food. With a Ghanaian mother you can see this being a problem as they love love love feeding people. My mom spends hours daily looking for foods and recipes that I might like. Looking for things that were a bit more flavourful to encourage me. The saddest day came when my family bought me a cinnzeo cinnamon bun (which is by far my favourite treat) with extra icing. I popped it in the microwave excitedly and started eating. I COULDN'T taste a thing. This shows the extent of my loss of taste buds. I remember crying because I just wanted to enjoy a meal for once rather than having to force feed high calorie meals to maintain weight.

My advice to you is please please please do not eat your favourite food during this time. You may regret it. Sometimes when you are force feeding yourself and then nauseated afterwards it changes how you feel about certain foods. The last thing you want is to associate your favourite foods with nausea. Smoothies used to be my go-to breakfast before transplant, it was a quick way to add calories to my day by blending up ensure and ice for a 300-calorie drink. But now I can't even look at a smoothie, let alone drink it. So just a warning! Like many other things in transplant finding foods that you can taste and enjoy is trial and error. When all else fails grate spicy cheese on everything, it worked for me maybe it will work for you!

Section C: Skin & Bone Changes

Bone Pain aka Engraftment

The first time I experienced this bone pain, I was convinced that the transplant didn't work and I was having a sickle cell crisis. The pain was mild but it startled me. I thought sickle cell disease was the only thing that could cause that deep deep bone aches and throbbing but I was wrong. Terrified I reported these findings to my transplant team and they smiled and were ecstatic, I looked at them like they must have misheard what I said. Then they filled me in and told me that what I am experiencing is getting first signs of engraftment, which means my sisters cells have made it to my bone marrow and were beginning to produce new cells. I just wondered why an event that was so joyous, had to be so painful. I was beginning to think that everything associated with transplant had to be painful.

If you've had a sickle cell crisis before you'll be able to easily deal with engraftment pain, discomfort and soreness. I was given Tylenol, Advil and narcotics to help control this pain. I would also recommend a heated blanket to wrap yourself in.

Skin Rashes, Dryness & Peeling

Pre-transplant they always talk about this idea of shedding your skin and discovering the new you, your new normal. I didn't realize that was literally what happened. I was shedding my skin like crazy. I was dry and peeling no matter how much lotion I put on. Have you ever dried yourself off after a shower and looked at your towel? My white towel was brown. My skin was literally shedding. I would put lotion on my legs and then one hour later it was like I haven't used lotion in days. I had dry scales all over my legs.

Then the rashes started, my entire face was covered in tiny little bumps for weeks and myself and my medical team couldn't figure out what it was. Then the bumps spread to my chest, and a few days later my back. At this point my medical team decided to do a skin biopsy to ensure that the bumps were not graft versus host disease (GVHD). Skin rashes and irritation are one of the many ways GVHD can rear its ugly head. Thankfully the biopsy did not show GVHD but it revealed a medication allergy.

So how do you deal with the skin changes? Keep your skin clean, so washing your face and showering daily. Your skin becomes so sensitive, so using milder soaps and unscented options help. Hydrate hydrate hydrate. I struggled to find a cream that actually kept my skin quenched, CeraVe body and face moisturizer worked really well for me. Glysomed and Cetaphil also are good options to test out. If none of that works let me know, I made a homemade shea butter cream that has transformed my skin and I'm happy to share!

Scalp Pain & Hair Loss

The scalp pain and soreness started a few days after radiation. Which makes sense since your entire body is being synched why wouldn't your head be affected as well. I had cornrows in my hair so I didn't notice that my hair was beginning to weaken/fall out until one day I looked in the mirror and saw that my edges had officially been snatched. At about four weeks post-transplant, it was time to take out my cornrows. I took out the extension and to my surprise I still had hair on my head after I finished, I even gave my hair a comb and I still had so much hair on my head. I thought I was immune to this hair loss I was warned about prior to transplant, all of this was true until I went to wash my hair. The moment the water touched my hair I knew something was wrong. The water hitting my hair sounded like water hitting metal roofing or plastic. I ignored it and continued with my wash routine, I put the shampoo in my hair and started rubbing in the roots. My fingers kept on getting stuck until I got to the point that my hair just turned into a ball that I could no longer work with. My eyes began swelling up with tears and I kept repeating to myself "Revée be strong". I turned off the shower water, dried myself and my knotted hair and called my mom. She was speechless and had no idea what she could even say that could potentially comfort me. I vividly remember Face-Timing my sister and my brother-in-law in tears. They showed up the next morning with a shaver and got to work. Since my hair was dry, brittle and only some of it decided to fall out, I opted to skip the trauma of watching it fall out and just to shave it now. The first time I looked at myself in the mirror after shaving my head was tough, but eventually I got used to this new normal and the look actually started to grow on me. In this situation I had to teach myself to focus on the positives, as much as I loved my long luscious hair, I began to enjoy the cool, high fashion edge this style gave me. So, my mom took me to the store when I was cleared and I bought a pair of hoop earrings to really complete the look. This was really a case of when life gives you lemons, you don't just stare at the lemons, you make lemonade or slice them and toss into your drink.

Before and after shaving my head, I would frequently experience random soreness on various areas of my head. It was painful at times just to lay my head down to sleep. This seems small but imagine how irritated you would be if you're exhausted and not feeling well but you can't even rest your head. There wasn't anything I could do for this, my transplant team just advised me that it is normal and will go away with time but they couldn't outline how long that would be. Let me just tell you this lingered on to at least two years post-transplant. I still have a few extremely sensitive places on my head. I don't have a solution for this issue other than choosing hair styles that don't pull your hair.

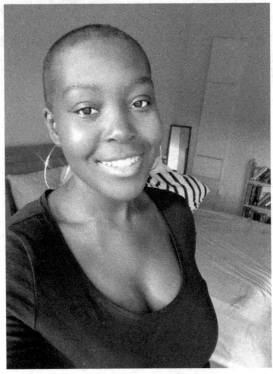

Section D: Sensory Changes

Tingling & Burning in Fingers

This symptom was very random but it developed about one-week post-transplant. Initially I just attributed it to an increase in the number of times I washed and sanitized my hands. I figured they were just dry. My hand would just start burning out of nowhere and I would apply lotion thinking that would help but it didn't make a difference. My transplant team advised me that there are some weird symptoms post-transplant that they can't always pinpoint what is causing it. Eventually after about a year this symptom disappeared thankfully.

Hallucinations

Man, these were bad. Hallucinations were the reason I was up every night until 2AM or 3AM hiding under my covers terrified. Hallucinations were also the reason I didn't want to get out of my bed to pee in the middle of the night. It sounds absolutely insane that a 25-year-old became afraid of the dark. I was told that my anti-rejection medication had the potential to cause some psychological and sensory disturbances but I didn't imagine it been quite like that. Let me tell you some of the crazy things I believed I was seeing. There was sky light in my bedroom in the condo, it was beautiful during the day but at night was a different story. The sky light needed to be replaced during my stay and the construction workers told us that it might take some time for the glass to "settle". What that really meant was that overnight when I was ready to get some sleep, I would hear so much creaking. For some reasons in my head that creaking was caused by little people in the room that were trying to pry open the glass so they could throw dirt at me and my immuno-compromised self. I was convinced that there were people trying to kill me. So, with thoughts like that every night you could see why I hid under my blankets. I don't even know how many mornings I would wake up and peek at the floor to make sure there wasn't dirt or dust on it. Then I'd ask my mom to vacuum the room for me. Thankfully being the great caregiver she was, she did it without questioning me. There wasn't really much that could be done about these but it lasted until my 100 days and then when I moved back to my house in Edmonton I actually felt fine. Maybe because my room at home didn't have a sky light ha-ha.

CHAPTER SIXTEEN

A FOODIES NIGHTMARE

You may or may not have already picked up on the fact that I'm a foodie. There is nothing I love more than eating my favourite food or sharing a nice meal with family and friends. So, transplant was a bother because I was so restricted with what I could eat. Oh, this is about to get really awkward if you're getting a transplant already and no one told you. There are lots of food related restrictions because you are immunocompromised after treatment. Meaning things will have to change.

A few ways your relationship with food will change:

- You are encouraged to eat small meals frequently to help keep it down due to the nausea you may experience.

- Eat high protein and calorie meals which to me really meant slather butter, cheese and soya sauce on everything (I did this before transplant but now I had an excuse).

- You are discouraged from eating out, of course because you don't know how sanitary things behind the prep desk really are. Think about it, what is the longest stretch of time you've gone without eating any fast foods or eating out at a restaurant? Even when you can return to eating out you are discouraged from eating raw sushi and eating at buffets.

- Try to avoid unpasteurized milk, cheese or yogurt, unwashed fruits and veggies, and unwashed salad. Even when I did eat any fruits or veggies, I washed them in a homemade diluted vinegar spray to ensure they were safe.

- You are encouraged to eat fresh food every day, growing up in an African home where we cooked large portions of stews, meats and soups then ate it all week this was going to be a challenge. We found a way around this by still cooking a medium sized amount of food, separating them into small meals in Tupperware and freezing a few days at a time. Then I could defrost and eat as needed.

You're probably thinking I am a drama queen because it doesn't seem like much but honestly when you're told you can't have something, you want it that much more. I think the combination of everything you are experiencing physically and mentally, then add on a full whack of food restrictions, can leave you feeling quite miserable. After some time, I got used to all of the restrictions and then it just became a way of life. I got used to the idea that I can't just go to a restaurant and get food. When you are deprived of something it's such a nice feeling to finally taste it again. It was nice to gradually introduce foods that I used to love back into my diet. A few foods that I was very excited about been reunited with were sushi and soft serve ice-cream! Even though the restriction process can be tough, it's worth it in the end!

If you're looking for high calorie meals that you can only get away with eating during transplant, I'm your girl.

Some of my favourites were:

- cinnamon buns
- pizza pockets with jalapeno cheese sprinkled on top
- homemade chili with extra cheese and sour cream
- homemade poutine and double the cheese
- rice and veggies loaded with steak sauce
- pizza and mozzarella sticks
- chicken burger and fries with gravy

My apologies if I just made you head to the pantry and grab an unhealthy snack. However, if you're struggling with weight gain, you can thank me later.

CHAPTER SEVENTEEN

MEDICATIONS "PILL POPPING"

After a while I was beginning to feel like my job during transplant was just to pop pills. When I was a kid, my parents had to hide my pills in rice for me to try and swallow them or crush them into juice. The younger me never would have imagined that I'd be downing six pills at a time with little to no water. I know people, miracles happen.

In the first 100 days post-transplant these were the medications that I was taking. Some were off and on, some were trial and error, and some the whole time.

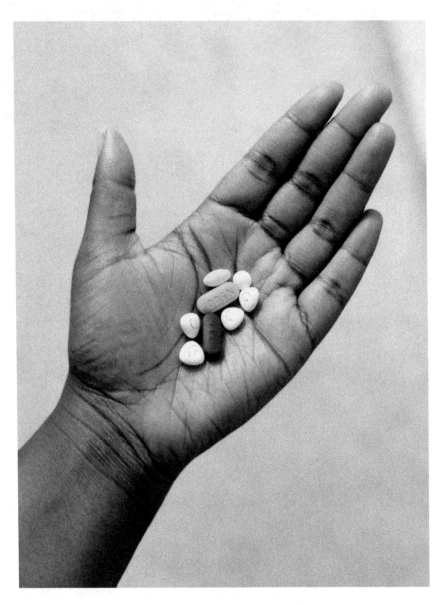

Here are my post-transplant medications in no particular order, trust me I haven't picked favourites!

Antirejection

Sirolimus

You could call this medication my life line. If you had any plans to skip a mediation this would be the last one. This medication is an anti-rejection/immunosuppression drug, meaning it kept my immune system at bay so my sister's cells had a chance to take the steering wheel.

Antibiotics

Penicillin

Septra

Dapsone

Cephalexin

These medications helped protect my body from bacterial infections.

Antiviral

Valacyclovir

This helped protect my body from viruses. When your immune system gets wiped out so does all of those years of immunizations. This medication protected me until I began immunizations about a year post-transplant and I didn't stop it until my live vaccinations at two years post-transplant.

Antifungal

Fluconazole

Yes, just like you can get bacterial or viral infections, you can also get fungal infections. This medication provided me with protection against that.

Narcotics/Pain Control

Morphine

Naproxen

These helps combat the bone pain and severe headaches I was experiencing.

Antiemetics

Zofran

Gravol

Maxeran

These medications were my life savers most days, they helped keep my nausea at bay.

Stomach Control

Lax-a-day (laxative)

This one helped me stay regular, I told you my insides were a mess so yup this was definitely needed.

Pantoprazole

This one helped control the amount of stomach acid I produced, helping reduce reflux and gastric pains.

Vitamins

Folic acid

This one helps you make red blood cells.

Other

Akabutu's mouthwash

THE BEST I repeat BEST mouthwash for chemo related mouth sores

Hydrocortisone cream

For all of the itchy skin rashes I developed

Pink lady mouthwash

Great spot treatment for mouth sores

Colchicine

An anti-inflammatory medication that helped me combat pericarditis

Benadryl cream and pills

For all of the itchiness

CHAPTER EIGHTEEN

MENTAL STRUGGLES

So, we've covered what the first 100 days looked like in terms of physical symptoms and some advice to combat those symptoms. I was semi prepared for the physical symptoms because you are warned about what transplant can do to your body, you have to be aware of these things in order to make an appropriate decision about transplant. But what is not often discussed in detail is the mental and emotional implications of transplant. This is something that I was not prepared for in any way shape or form. I knew that physical transplant would be difficult but I knew sickle cells had prepared me to deal with the physical pain and symptoms I might come against.

Section A: Isolation

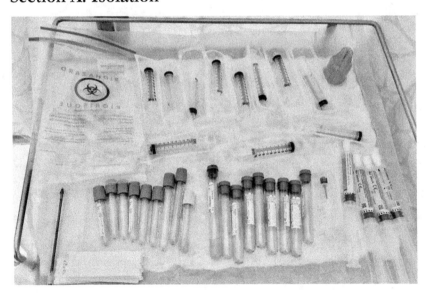

So why is transplant so emotionally draining? I'll give you a few reasons.

Physical Isolation

Because you are at so much risk, you have to create physical distance between your friends, family and coworkers. In my case I live in Edmonton and the transplant was done in Calgary which is three hours away. So, the distance made it even harder to be surrounded by those you love. My mom stayed with me in Calgary and my dad would come up every other weekend, my boyfriend every weekend, my sister every few weeks when she had the opportunity and my brother made it up to visit as well. But these visits were often cancelled if the person was feeling unwell. I felt like a burden on my family because they would work during the week, be tired on the weekend like everyone else and then have to drive three hours for a short visit before it was time for them to turn back and do it all over again. I carried a significant amount of guilt during this time. Even when they came, after a while I noticed everyone seemed to have a mild level of fear surrounding being around me. Everyone wanted to find the perfect balance between close but not too close, and hugging me tight enough to show me they missed me but not too tight that my fragile body would crumble. We'd all sit on the couch but no-one wanted to sit too close to me in case the off chance that they had a bug that their immune system could handle and mine couldn't. To ensure I was protected my family and I enforced very strict rules surrounding my visiting policy. Obviously if you were sick or was in the same household as anyone that was sick you weren't able to visit. Also, if you didn't have your flu shot, unfortunately you couldn't visit either. We decided it's better to be over cautious and keep me safe rather than regretting how relaxed we were if I got sick. Even my niece, who is afraid of everything medical, was brave enough to get her flu shot because she knew she had to be healthy to see her auntie. Now that's dedication!

Social Isolation

Also known as watching the world keep moving without you aka fear of missing out (FOMO). We've all stayed in from a birthday party and then had to sit through a whole week of everyone talking around you about all of the fun that they had, memories made and or course inside jokes that seemed to carry on for weeks. This idea or feeling of missing out is something that we've been experiencing since we were children asking for a toy that everyone else has and parents saying no. In my experience I found transplant an extremely trying time in the sense that it provided you with a lot of time to think. Which in some cases can be a good thing but in others it can be a bad one? At the time I was 25/26, so just like the majority of people around that age you're starting to realize you're not "young" anymore. I was wrapped up in this idea that since I am dating someone for over two years at the time, we should be thinking of our future together and making plans for that. I sat back and watched some of my closest friends, move in with partners, get engaged, plan weddings and some welcome babies into the world. It's natural to feel left out when it feels like your life is on hold but everyone else is still moving forward. Comparison truly is the thief of joy. I had to find a balance between listening to my friends tell me about all of the advancements in their lives and protecting my own mental health.

Funny enough on the other side my friends felt the same way. Majority of the people I would interact with had no idea how to approach me, based on their fear of saying the wrong thing. It's like when someone loses a loved one and you spend hours trying to figure out the perfect thing that will brighten their day but in reality, all they want to know is that you care. There isn't anything you can say to change their situation but support and feeling loved. My friends would often only ask about me and what things I've been experiencing but leave out their lives. I would commonly get the "awe I'm so sorry to hear that", "OMG that's so tough, I can't believe you're going through that" or "you're so strong". I appreciate their concern but sometimes I truly ran out of steam and was so tired of being "strong". I just wanted to be weak. Sometimes when I spoke to friends there was awkwardness because I felt tired of telling them about my sad life and they were scared to tell me about how great their life was.

It took some work but eventually we got to a place where people realized I did want to hear about the outside world and have "normal" conversations about work, family and men of course. I think finding that happy medium is important, but really, it's up to you to figure out what that happy medium looks like to you. Just remember that you have to put yourself first and make the decision. Do not let others decide for you. I think this rule applies to many areas of life, we often want to be so accommodating to others but then forget our own needs and wants in the process.

Section B: Mind Games

Anxiety & Worry

Oh yeah, I feel like this one should be a no brainer. Transplant or any medical encounter can be really scary and cause a fair amount of stress, anxiety and worry. In my case, transplant was very scary because I was about to be the first adult in Alberta and maybe even in Canada to be transplanted for sickle cell disease. At that point I knew many other adults had been transplanted for sickle cells in the United Kingdom (UK) and United States of America (USA). What worried me is that my dedication and persistence landed me in the role of guinea pig or I guess a better word is ground breaker. Transplant aside every time I entered a hospital, I felt like there was always a level of the unknown that was just right around the corner. With a typical sickle cell pain crisis, you could spend 24 hours in the emergency, two days on an inpatient unit or two weeks. Sickle cells was always very unpredictable to me, you could do everything in your power to ensure that you avoid "triggers" and still end up in a pain crisis. There was always a sense of anxiety in terms of what physician you would get, would they truly believe you were in pain or just assume you were drug seeking? So, prior to transplant I was already no stranger to uncertainty, anxiety and worry. With transplant it felt different, it felt scarier because it was something I wasn't familiar with. I felt like I was going in blind. I liked to be well researched before I do any type of medical procedure but well researching transplant just left me in tears. When you search for transplant all you find are pages and pages of symptoms and adverse side effects. That would definitely make a person not want to be an expert in all things transplant because you'd spend your days obsessing over all of the possible issues you could run into. So, I knew enough to be aware and spot warning signs if things seemed off but that's about it. I didn't try and learn all of the things that may go wrong years later, because that's just stressful. My advice to you is to know what to expect and be aware of things to watch for. Don't bury yourself in stories, articles and medical journals.

My anxiety and worry also stemmed from a place of constantly being on high alert. Because this was uncharted territory it was important that you were attentive to seemingly mild things that could turn into something bad. I took note of everything I ate every day, and any symptom I experienced that day and then charted it in my transplant binder. This binder became a communication tool for me that helped me explain to my transplant team what was going on. Sounds like a great idea but when you are constantly "on duty" and watching for possible issues you don't allow yourself to relax. No way you give yourself one hour free of stress and worry, you could miss something and die! Right?! All of this worry started pouring into other areas of my life. Rather than just being stressed about transplant my mind decided to play tricks on me and permitted me to also stress about my future. Because one thing wasn't enough? I would often find myself lying in bed spending so much time wondering if everything I've worked for up until this point was all for nothing, because the intrusive thought that I may never make it out of Calgary clouded my thoughts.

Disappointment

Oh, disappointment was probably the one that hit me the hardest. Go through a huge medical event and trust me your true friends will reveal themselves. As well as some people you though could care less about you would somehow pop out of the woodwork ready to support you. Most people who know me know that I do not like asking for help. I am very much a do it yourself, independent woman. Transplant forced me to lean on people which was something I was never comfortable doing nor did I enjoy doing. I liked to support myself because sometimes when you lean on others or set expectations that gives people the power to disappoint you. And trust me that's exactly what happened. So, in the real world you see some of your closer friends weekly, every other week or maybe okay at most once a month. Imagine how let down you might feel when you've been in Calgary undergoing a life changing treatment that you could potentially die from, it's day 68 and some of your closest friends hadn't made the effort to come and see you. That may sound extremely self-centered for me to say. In reality I was suffering and that's when I truly needed my friends, I needed support. I was constantly overwhelmed with the thought that I might not make it out, so naturally it really hurt to feel like your friends knew that and still couldn't make you a priority. It made me feel like a lot of people only surrounded themselves with me because I was "fun" but when I wasn't fun anymore and things got serious, they ran for the hills. But on the opposite side, you'd be surprised by the people who maybe weren't in your inner circle but showed up for you more than ever. I had friends that I only spoke to twice a year previously that made it their mission to brighten my day. I'll go into the kindness I experience more in detail later.

Disturbed Sleep Patterns

Something that really had me on edge was my disturbed sleep patterns. When you can't sleep you can't function, period. You're miserable the next day so everything that you experience feels like doomsday. My crazy nighttime hallucinations that were keeping me up all night. After a while the lack of sleep does take a toll on you. It didn't make sense to me how someone who was home all day and night, didn't have any responsibilities and spent most of the day in bed had bags under their eyes. Oh, that someone was me. Asides from the hallucinations another really big issue was the endless flow of medications. Some of my medications were drowsy so I'd take it at 4PM and then get so tired and take a nap late afternoon keeping me up all night. I turned to melatonin to try and help me sleep at night but I was finding that the dose just kept increasing and I still wasn't really getting any sleep. My doctor suggested meditation, I looked at him like he was crazy because I was seriously wondering what meditation would do for me. I was desperate and willing to try anything, so I downloaded one of those meditation apps and to my surprise it was amazing. It helped me relax before bed and focus on my breathing rather than staring up at the sky light terrified. I urge anyone that is struggling with sleep regardless of the cause to at least trial meditation, you might be as pleasantly surprised as I was.

CHAPTER NINETEEN

THE BEAUTY WITHIN TRANSPLANT

I feel like the previous section scared you away from transplant and made you feel like it's just traumatic. Okay, yes, it can be traumatic at some points but it also was wonderful in so many ways. Let me explain.

The outpouring of love that I experienced was amazing. I think health scares have the potential to bring out the best in people. People are inherently good and they love to help. This outpouring of love started even before I went to Calgary. I mentioned earlier that God sent a woman that was kind enough to allow myself and my family a place to stay during transplant. Kindness like I had never experienced before. I was preparing to pay $1500 monthly for hospital apartment accommodation that wasn't old and dingy. Instead, I was blessed with an immaculate two-bedroom, two-bathroom top floor condo that overlooked the bow river! Throughout the duration of my time in Calgary she made it her mission to find ways to brighten my day, with check in phone calls and food drop offs. After encountering her I was and will always be forever changed. She makes me want to pay it forward and find ways to help others the best I can.

There was some disappointment related to how some of my friends reacted to my transplant but there were also lots of surprises - acts of kindness from my friends. On multiple occasions my sister and niece would surprise me with a visit when they knew things were getting rough, I didn't even have to ask them to come, it was just automatic. My boyfriend at the time stayed up until 3AM some nights to help me through my hallucinations. I had a friend cook meal for my boyfriend because they empathized with the fact that he probably didn't have much time to take care of himself as he spent every day off driving to see me. I had a friend from work that sent me a meme she knew I'd like every single day, just to make me smile. Pregnant friends that showed up bearing gifts and had a smile on their face even though they spent three hours in a car throwing up. Friends that organized impromptu game nights and fancy breakfasts. Friends that spend the entire weekend making me laugh and cracking jokes. A friend that facetimed me pretty much every day even though she herself was hospitalized but still found a way to pencil me in. A friend with a small child that made the drive multiple times, despite how hard it may be to drive three hours with a one-year-old. Cousins that drove down to see me and brought so many of my favourite foods and childhood snacks. I had a family friend that lived in Calgary who came to visit me every week and we would watch trash TV together, it felt so nice to feel "normal" and just have a hang out. I'm telling you; people love to help; you just have to allow them!

CHAPTER TWENTY

MY CAREGIVER

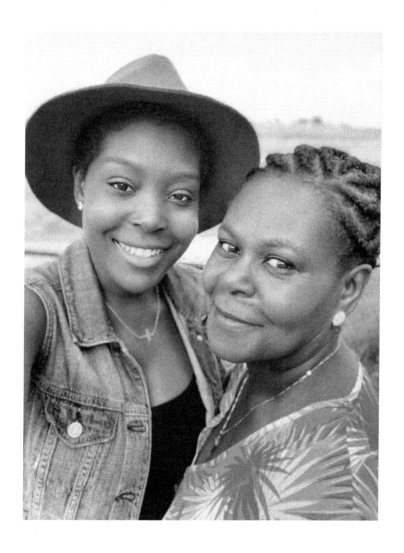

"To be a caregiver you have to be able to put on a brave face, smile and make jokes all day so the person you're caring for will smile too. You can't take away their pain but you can at least make them smile for a minute and forget their worries" – Mom.

My mom during this time had to be my caregiver and she really and truly put her own life completely on hold for me. Just imagine how that would make you feel that someone was willing to pack up for the call of duty to be there for you. We had some tough times because trust me it's not easy spending 24 hours a day cooped up in a suite for months with the same person. No matter how much you love and care about the person. Spending so much time together will definitely put you on edge. We became very proficient at finding things to argue about. Some days we didn't talk much and things were strictly business (ensuring I was feeling okay and taking medications) and other days we would go on walks down the bow river, chatting and enjoying the views. There is no such thing as a perfect caregiver and as a patient you have to understand that. No one is going to say or do all of the things you want at the right time. I honestly wished I realized this while I was in Calgary because my mom and I would have had a more positive experience together. At the time I didn't really see how much my mom was doing for me and that was truly my own ignorance and self-centeredness.

There's no class on how to be a good caregiver, there's no guide on the right things to say when supporting someone through a tough time, and there's no book on the perfect balance of show-ing concern and allowing space. My mom was doing her best but I barely saw it. Every morning she would peek into my room to make sure I was doing okay; she cooked every single meal I'd asked for and at times even cooked a second or third meal if I couldn't taste the food or it wasn't sitting well. She would help me stay on schedule with my medications, bring them for me if I wasn't able or didn't feel like getting up. She would fix bath water to the per-fect temperature and even bathe me if I asked (I never did but I know she would in a heartbeat). If the fatigue was really bad and I couldn't even get dressed, she would find the clothes I selected and then dress me as I sat limp on the bed. She stripped my bed for me every other day and washed all of the laundry. She did all of the daily cleaning and deep cleaning for me. Despite all she did for me, we would argue often and there was friction but the one thing that would always bring us back together was the Ellen Show that came on daily at 4PM. The Ellen show was like our escape, it gave us a break and something light hearted and funny to bond over and enjoy together. I was in my own little world and so focused on all of the things that were not going as planned, rather than focusing on the things that were going right. The transplant team is adamant that anyone who gets a stem cell transplant needs a caregiver or won't perform the treatment, so really if I didn't have my mom as a caregiver the transplant may not have happened. I am so thankful she was able to support me through this process. Thank your caregivers for everything they do for you. I mean that even in terms of when you are sick at home with a cold or the stomach flu, the person that is checking on you, refreshing your drink and bringing you meals. I think sometimes we all forget that people have a choice, and if they choose to help, we need to appreciate them and show gratitude.

It's important to choose the right caregiver to support you through transplant or any health journey. Below I outlined some of the tasks that your caregiver may have to do for you, so ensure they are willing to do so, as well as ensure you are comfortable with doing those things. During transplant you will be at your most vulnerable state so you will need someone that is attentive, cares deeply about your wellbeing and someone that you are comfortable with. Choosing the right person to stand by your side will make all the difference.

"Being a caregiver is very rewarding knowing that you are supporting someone you love and care about. However, being a caregiver was also the most stressful and scary thing that I ever had to do. I lived in a constant state of fear, worrying about every little thing that I did. Hoping that I didn't make a mistake that would cost my daughter her life" – Mom.

Below are some tips my mom wanted me to share with you. These are some of the things that she did while being my caregiver. These are in no way shape or form mandatory; we're just sharing some things that worked for us. Please consult your transplant team for your specific guidelines and instructions.

Tips From One Caregiver To Another

The Basics

- Carry an emergency bag! Mine included a small first aid kit, emergency PICC line dressing supplies, mask, gloves, sanitizer, my daughters' medications and of course her binder of hospital information that went everywhere with us.

- Program the transplant clinics information into your phone or have their contact information handy.

- Remember the medications the person you are caring for is taking and when they are expected to be given, so you can provide reminders and help keep them on track.

- Try to be creative, look for games and things you guys can do to pass time.

- Understand that the person you're caring for isn't feeling well and they will be leaning on you not only physically but emotionally. At times you may be their punching bag or their shoulder to cry on but you're also the person that can bring them joy when they need it most.

Keeping Things Clean

- Have hand sanitizer with you at all time. The person you're caring for might need it. This should be easy now since we just lived through a global pandemic.

- Wash your hands every time you enter the home and ensure anyone that comes to visit also does the same. The person you're caring for will have a weakened immune system and can have a harder time fighting off infections.

- Daily bathroom cleaning and kitchen cleaning with bleach and other disinfectants became a routine. (If you are sharing a bathroom with the person, you're caring for it's best to give everything you touch a quick disinfect after each use).

- Change the bedding minimum every three days. If not, the entire bedding changing pillow cases that can harbour bacteria frequently is important.

Food

- Wash all fruits and veggies in a diluted vinegar rinse to ensure they are clean and safe to eat.

- Cook food in small portions so that it doesn't go bad. I ensured any food that my patient would be eating only stayed in the fridge for 24 hours. Anything that wouldn't be eaten in 24 hours was frozen and defrosted as she needed.

- You have to be okay with cooking multiple meals daily because it is likely that the person you are caring for isn't eating the same food as you.

Last by not least. sleep with one eye open because you don't want to miss anything. Just joking. Get good rest because you have to take care of yourself first to ensure you can adequately care for someone else.

CHAPTER TWENTY-ONE

A NEW OUTLOOK

Myself First & Priority

I've always been a giver; I've always been the person that despite how bad I feel I get up and tend to a friend in need. I often cause myself stress trying to be there for everyone through their hard times and forget how important it is for me to take care of myself. During transplant I really started to learn and implement the importance of putting myself first and making my needs a priority. Essentially, I learned how to "get selfish." There are times in life to give but there are also times in life to receive. So that's exactly what I did, I stopped making decisions based on guilt and obligation but rather on how I felt. This school of thought hit me when I started realizing that regardless of me getting a transplant the world around me was still moving. People were still going to parties, my best friends were still hanging out without me, trips were still being booked and relationships were still progressing. If everyone was still living their best life despite what I was dealing with, it's time for me to start living how I wanted to live and stop catering to others. It was refreshing to say no to a phone conversation when I knew I needed some time to pray. It was nice to decide if the days visitors wanted to come worked for me rather than automatically saying yes. It was nice to reply to a text the next day because I had a late-night bath and needed some me time. I stopped allowing others to schedule my day and rather began to schedule them into my life. I chose the conversations I wanted to have and the people I wanted to spend my time with. I am so glad I learned this during my time in Calgary because it became increasingly important once I was back in Edmonton. You need to care for yourself before you care for others. Remember life goes on regardless of what you choose, so you might as well choose what's best for you!

Something that also ties into making yourself a priority is developing your skills and learning about yourself. I learned so much about myself during this time. I learned more about myself during transplant than I did up until that point. I took time to perfect my knitting skills, learn how to cook some new meals, develop a brand that would eventually surge me into new opportunities. This was a time for self-discovery and I loved it! I've always been a go getter but I didn't realize how much I could withstand. Transplant pushed me to my absolute limits and to be able to continually motivate myself to keep going was something I never knew I could do. It gave me a new sense of confidence that I can do absolutely anything I put my mind to. This is why the scripture "I can do all things through Christ who strengthens me" Philippians 4:13 became my life line.

Leaning On God

The most important thing I learned while in Calgary was to trust God. It sounds simple and you probably feel like I should have already been trusting in God. Let me clarify, it's not that I wasn't trusting of God before but the way I had to lean on Him was something I've never encountered before. Everyone freely says they are trusting God when things are good but when things get bad, do we still trust Him? Can we still trust Him? Honestly my relationship with God has been rocky since the day I researched sickle cell disease at age 12 and the life expectancy was 14. I couldn't comprehend how a loving God would give me such a "curse"; it just didn't make sense to me. I suffered year after year, felt my body get weaker and weaker, allowed my mental health to get worse and worse and eventually my relationship with God became more and more distant. But transplant turned things around for me. I was going to face a treatment that no one else I knew had ever done, it would be a first for the doctors, I would be a guinea pig. I was going in blind but I knew God could see what the future held for me. I went in with the thought that if I die, at least I know my experience will help someone else be that much closer to their cure. At least the doctors would know what not to do the next time around. I was terrified of the unknown so all I could do was lean on God and truly believe that He knows exactly what He was doing. Almost every night I cried out to Him, thanked Him for bringing me to the point I am at, thanked Him for the opportunity in front of me and fully yielded all to Him. His will was the only way and I knew that. Every new symptom I experienced all I could do was hand it over to God and ask for Him to strengthen me as I endured. To my surprise every side effect that came at me, eventually passed. None took me down or made me quit. Trust me there were days I wanted to quit but I asked God for strength and the grace to keep pushing forward. It was interesting because God was my guide but He never audibly spoke to me, He just opened the doors in the directions He wanted me to go. So, when a door opened, I knew it was for a reason. I wish I would have known all of this going into transplant and not come to the realization afterwards.

I felt so alone and isolated during transplant. I felt like there was no one in the world who could really understand how horrible I felt mentally and physically. People would try and comprehend but I still felt this distance between us. I sit back now and realize that God was doing this on purpose. He was pushing people away because He knew if they stayed close, I would lean on them and put my trust in them, which will only lead to disappointment. God wanted to show me that He was there for me. God was there during the late-night hallucinations, during the days my head was held over a toilet, during the days I couldn't get out of bed, during the days my bones ached, during the times my heart yearned for someone to understand, He was there and He understood it all. I truly believe that God intentionally allowed me to experience every single side effect and negative symptom because He knew that I would be sitting in my kitchen today and writing this book. It didn't make sense at the time but now I see it clearly. God had a plan and He always will have a plan for your life. In the midst of chaos, it seems impossible to take the time and really understand what God is doing for you. Oftentimes, it's after the event we sit back and realize that God did it again without us even knowing it. So, I handed my life over to God, sat back and watched Him guide my steps, treatments, recovery and take me to greater heights. Lean on Him, embrace Him and see what happens.

CHAPTER TWENTY-TWO

ANSWERED PRAYERS

January 25, 2018

I woke up today like any other clinic day. At this point my clinic visits had been reduced from daily, to every other day to twice a week to now weekly Thursday appointments. The previous Thursday I had a skin biopsy taken from a rash that started on my face, spread to my chest and then eventually my back and shoulders. I won't lie, I was terrified for those results. The team did the biopsy to figure out if the rash was potentially a GVHD of the skin. Getting these results really would declare the beginning of the end and that's what I was expecting. Ironic that I just spent a whole chapter talking about my renewed faith in God but we are only human, as faith filled as I felt I still had my anxieties. I got ready with my mom that morning and we headed over to the hospital. I sat in the BMT waiting room filling out the questionnaire that asked you to rank yourself on a scale of 1-10 for various categories like appetite, fatigue, nausea, anxiety, depression and overall wellbeing. At that precise moment I wanted to rank myself at 10/10 on the anxiety scale. I was startled when the nurse called my name and we walked through the clinic doors into our treatment room. After waiting for what felt like forever my physician came in and we discussed how the week has been. I opened up my big binder with my daily tick chart like the real nerd I am and reviewed day by day some of the things I was experiencing. For the most part I was doing great, it was just the anxiety that was getting to me. In my mind I just kept on thinking "can he cut to the chase, what are the results!" Then finally the moment of truth.

He started with "well Revée good news for you". Once he said that my stress immediately lifted. He told me that my biopsy results were negative for GVHD. He told me that the rash was likely due to an allergy to Penicillin. I would take a penicillin reaction over GVHD any day. So, my doctor decided to change my antibiotic and then just like that the problem was solved. I felt like I could finally breathe again. Felt like a weight was lifted off my shoulders.

Then he said "wait there's more," he proceeded to tell me that since I have been feeling so well for the most part, I should start preparing myself for discharge. I was a bit confused at first because I was already discharged from the hospital but what he meant was discharged from the Calgary BMT team because they were getting ready to send me home! I was told that for sure by my 100 days post-transplant I would be back home. I was ecstatic, I couldn't believe that my time in Calgary was coming to an end. Strange enough I was so excited to leave but at the same time I was afraid of being away from my transplant team. Yes, there would be another team in Edmonton that would take care of me but they didn't know me and I didn't know them but I guess this was what I wanted. I was going to be that much closer to my new normal. My mom began thanking God for this amazing news. At this point we were so excited and already planning our celebratory meal for later that evening.

Then very casually he said, "oh Revée here are your lab results from earlier this morning. By this time, he knew me so well and knew that I documented all of the lab results in my trusty binder. Since the beginning of transplant, the team has closely been monitoring my white blood cells (infection fighting cells), red blood cells (oxygen carrying cells) and my platelets (blood clotting cells). Over the weeks we watched all my numbers plummet from the chemo and radiation then the exciting part began. We got to watch all of my numbers increase indicating that my sister's cells made it into my bone marrow and was doing its work. Essentially what that means is that the transplant is working as planned. After all the blood, sweat and tears that I've endured in the past few months there was nothing better than hearing that. We also watched my sickled hemoglobin, the number of sickled red blood cells floating around in my bloodstream. The higher the sickled hemoglobin the more likely you are to experience the complications of sickle cell disease. Going into my final red cell exchange one week before my transplant admission, my sickle hemoglobin (Hgb S) was 55%, after the treatment it was down to 35%. Over the months I watched it decline to 17%, 8% and then eventually to 4%. I couldn't believe it; I've never lived a life with only 4% sickled cells in my body. I was excited for life with no pain and worries. Then my doctor handed me my results from this morning. I examined the paper and the moment I saw it my eyes welled up with tears. Across from Hgb S it said NEGATIVE. I was officially sickle cell free! I looked at mom and was like, "mom I don't have sickle cells anymore?" I was in shock and I didn't even fully understand the weight of the words I was saying. My mom jumped up and started cheering! We hugged my doctor and he congratulated me. I was in awe and total disbelief. I felt stunned and confused because when I thought of transplant, I knew that the goal was to cure sickle cell disease but I just didn't realize until that moment that curing sickle cell disease really and truly meant, I no longer had any detectable sickle cells in my body. That afternoon we went home on a high, we couldn't even comprehend what we just heard. It was one thing to find out that I was GVHD negative, another thing to find out that I'm doing well enough to start preparing for discharge from Calgary but this, finding out I was officially sickle cell free was too much! We praised and thanked God. Every second word that came out of my mouth was "Thank You Jesus". I honestly don't think I stopped crying for days because I was truly so happy. As happy and joyful as I was there was a part of me that was hesitant to be too happy, that little seed of doubt in the back of mind made me question if this was just a fluke and the next test would say positive. But I forced myself to stay positive because deep down I knew God had already ordained my healing so all I needed to do was accept it. It's funny how when we get exactly what we want sometimes we question it because it seems too good to be true. This wasn't too good to be true, it was just true. It was surreal and honestly still surreal to this day. I never imagined a life without sickle cells and I never had any idea what that would look like and now I was being given the opportunity to experience life with less restrictions, life with less fear, and live where I can be confident that I can achieve anything. There hasn't been a single day since January 25, 2018 that I haven't thanked God for what he has done for me. I am in awe of God's love for me and you should be too. Imagine one of the first prayers I remember praying as a child has been answered. I used to laugh and get irritated when my parents told me that I was one day going to get cured. Because in my small faithless mind I didn't think it was possible, I felt I was option less. But 15 years later God still answered. I use this experience as a benchmark of God's love, grace and blessings upon my life. If He can cure me from an incurable disease with a life expectancy of 14 years, He can do anything. Now I am sitting here writing this book at age 29 sickle cell free and with a traumatic story that became a testimony. If God can do this, He can do anything. If He can do this for me, He can do it for you. Whether you have a chronic illness that's left you feeling hopeless, a family situation that pains you, a job promotion that won't seem to come, a school exam that you just can't pass. Know that God is with you and He will see you through it.

CHAPTER TWENTY-THREE

DISCHARGED

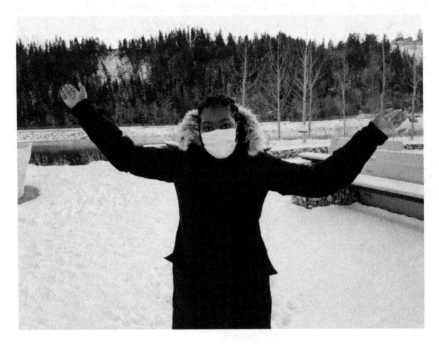

J ust like that we were packing the last bits of our things into the car and saying goodbye to the condo which became our tempo-rary home. With tears in my eyes, I thanked the condo owner for the kindness and generosity she showed me and my family, I know that without her my transplant experience wouldn't have been so positive. I reassured her that her kindness won't stop with me and that I will ensure I pay it forward to others. After a tearful goodbye we got into the car and I was watching Calgary fade away while Edmonton grew closer.

When I got home, I was welcomed by balloons from my brother with a beautiful message and a fully redecorated room by my sister and brother-in-law. I was so happy to be home and even happier that my family was excited to have me back. Although I was home now there was a sense of insecurity, surrounding my ability to keep myself safe and maintain the same standard of isolation/disinfection. It was nice to be back in my domain, in a place I felt fully comfortable. I was excited to live the life after transplant that I was promised, there were so many unknowns ahead but at least I was getting a second chance at life.

CHAPTER TWENTY-FOUR

SHOULDN'T I BE HEALTHY NOW?

I guess this was my own fault but I was under the impression that
been discharged from the Calgary BMT team meant that I was
"better now", "healthy", "ready to get back to life". NOPE, I was
certainly wrong. Discharge from Calgary merely meant I was going
home to continue my recovery. I was still supposed to be isolating,
I was still taking the same meds, I was still eating based on the same
guidelines, I was still fatigued all the time, I was still experiencing
some of the side effects of transplant and yes, I was still anxious
sometimes about something going wrong. It felt like I was home but
not really. I think being distant from family and friends was hard
when I was in Calgary but then I realized that being distant from
family and friends when you are only 20 minutes away from them
was even harder. It felt like I was living on the outside still. I had to
be cautious of the people that I allowed into my space and ensure
they were healthy. My days were also filled with appointments so at
times I would be so exhausted when I returned home that I couldn't
see anyone even if I wanted to. I never went to anyone else's house
because I was afraid of catching a bug or something. Maybe I took
the paranoia to a new level but I wanted to be as safe as possible, I
made it this far so I was determined to come out of this experience
scot free.

A transplant misconception that I fell victim to was the thought
that having a transplant meant I would be instantly healthy. Before
transplant I know my physicians did say that it can take up to a

year for you to begin to feel like yourself again. For some reason I assumed that I was an exception to the rule and I would feel better right away since after all my nickname was "bionics". The first few weeks back home were rough because I was expecting a miraculous recovery. Kind of like when you are admitted to the hospital and get discharged after an extended amount of time you typically need some time to recover at home before you can get back to your "normal" duties. The nausea I had in Calgary was still lingering, the fatigue was still so prominent that climbing up the stairs to the bathroom would leave me exhausted, and the feeling of my life being on hold was still a thought that I recently had to battle with.

What people need to understand is that transplant is not a quick fix to cure sickle cells. Yes, you may be sickle cell free at the end but there is a whole load of transplant side effects that you will be battling. Really, it's an exchange, you are exchanging one chronic illness for another. Yeah, I know that sounds kind of sad but you just need to decide which chronic illness you would rather have. I chose to be a stem cell transplant patient because it's better than living in constant pain. With both of these there was still a level of fear associated with the unknown. With sickle cells I was always worried about overdoing it and getting a pain crisis at an inopportune time leading to further bone, joint and organ damage. Post-transplant I was worried about catching a virus or bacteria that my developing immune system couldn't fight or getting GVHD that could slowly take over my body. I knew all of this before making my decision to go forward but there is a difference between hearing about what life would be like and truly living it. Being sickle cell free doesn't mean that you are free of all sickle cell related issues either. Being sickle cell free means that you no longer have sickle cells in your body causing damage but the damage that has already been done remains the same. So, the chronic knee pain I was already experiencing didn't go away, if anything some things worsened because of the effects of chemotherapy and radiation. It was liberating to return my collection of narcotics to pharmacy but at the same time I was picking up a whole plethora of other medications.

Medications that I was on when I returned to Edmonton were:

- Sirolimus 3mg (anti-rejection)

- Folic acid 5mg

- Vitamin D 1000 IU

- Valacyclovir 500mg (anti-viral)

- Colchicine 0.5mg twice a day (anti-inflammatory)

- Claritin (anti-itch)

- Cephalexin 500mg twice a day (antibiotic)

- Dapsone 25mg (antibiotic)

As you can see leaving Calgary, I also left with a bag full of medications and prescriptions, but on the bright side at least I was leaving Calgary!

A week after my return to Edmonton I had my first appointment at the Cross Cancer Institute. I was finally going to meet the Edmonton BMT team. My new physician, nurse and pharmacist all seemed very nice so I was happy to be in good hands. They didn't know much about sickle cell disease because their specialty was in oncology, nor have they had a sickle cell transplant patient but they seemed very willing to take on my care. I would meet with them every month for a clinic appointment where I could discuss concerns and they would track my progress. I was a bit weary because they didn't have an after-hours or on call number. So really, I could only reach them Monday to Friday from 8AM to 4PM, and if I ran into issues outside of that window, I would have to go to the emergency room. This thought scared me because in Calgary it was "beat into my head" that I shouldn't go to the emergency, as I am at higher risk for infections and emergency rooms are infection pools. I was advised to call the BMT physician on call after hours or during the day to call the clinic. I understand that was within my first 100 days, but my neutrophils (infection fighting cells) haven't really increased since I left. I just had to be hopeful that I was going to remain healthy and wouldn't have to go to the emergency.

CHAPTER TWENTY-FIVE

BUMPS IN THE ROAD

Transplant is like being on a rollercoaster. We've all been in the lineup of a rollercoaster ride and continually second guess if you can handle it. People tell you it will be scary but you'll be fine. So, you get on the rollercoaster, excited and nervous at the same time. Anticipation builds as you slowly approach the top. The first drop happens and you survive it so you're hoping that was the worst of it. You know there is a moment where you will go upside down but you just can't see it yet. Coming back to Edmonton felt like that, it felt like I was just waiting for the moment that I would be spun upside down.

The First Bump: Methemoglobinemia

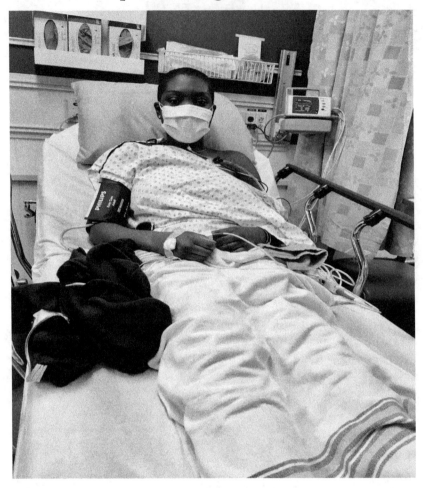

I had one of the best days I've ever had since transplant. I spend the day running around with my niece and nephew throwing snowballs and making snow men. It made me feel normal again, I felt like I could be the kids' auntie again, not this sick patient they constantly had to visit in the hospital. After running around all day having fun, I was exhausted by the evening and took some time to rest and even having an easy bed time was feeling so wiped. I woke up the next morning feeling a bit more fatigued than I usually do. I was annoyed because I thought I was supposed to be getting better not worse. I figured I likely over exerted myself the day before and just needed to take some time to rest. I anticipated after a bit of rest the next few days I would be back to normal. But the opposite happened, as the days progressed, I began feeling worse. The fatigue was intensifying and even going up the stairs became a feat. Moving from sitting or lying positions to standing meant I would be dizzy and could feel my heart beating rapidly. I was having piercing headaches that brought on nausea. All of my joints were achy before I even got out of my bed for the day. I had chills despite being wrapped up in a heated blanket. I would take a shower and find that I was short of breath and had to sit on the edge of the tub mid shower. I had a dry cough that with every cough intensified all of my other symptoms. I knew something wasn't right but I just couldn't seem to figure out what my body was trying to tell me.

I had a scheduled appointment with my transplant team on Monday so I waited it out till then. On Monday, I could barely walk. I was so exhausted, so with my mom holding my arm up I dragged myself into the Cross Cancer Institute. Once in the exam room with the team I explained my symptoms again in greater detail, because you know I wrote down everything that was going on day by day in usual Revée fashion. When I got to the exam room, I explained the symptoms I was having. At the time I was told that the symptoms were very broad that they were thinking I likely just over exhausted myself and my body now takes longer to bounce back from things that once didn't affect me. I was told the symptoms should resolve in no time. The nurse took my vitals, and for some weird reason my saturation probe was not working and it kept showing 85%-90%. For anyone that is not familiar with normal oxygenation the target range is 95%-100% but it depends on the person and what their baseline is. For me I knew my baseline was about 95% post-transplant so it was odd that my reading was so low. It was chalked up to be due to nail polish (side note I wasn't wearing any nail polish). For some reason it never occurred to any of the professionals in the room that maybe the reading was accurate. The physician, nurse and pharmacist discussed that they felt my symptoms were all secondary to stress since I just came back from Calgary and I was having trouble adjusting. So, I was given a prescription for massage and encouraged to take a hot bath when I got home. I was furious because I knew my body and I knew that this was not stress related. I know when I am stressed and was definitely not stressed, them not believing me was actually now causing me stress. I tried my best to accept their advice and at least take it easy for a few days, hoping that everything was going to turn around. It didn't so what do you think I did? You should know me by now I am extremely persistent and when I know something is off trust me, I will pursue it. So, I called the team back when I realized that I was getting worse rather than better. They brought me to the clinic to run some tests, I had a chest x-ray, an NP swab (if you don't know what that is, it's the longest swab that goes up your nose and I swear into your brain ha-ha at least that's what it felt like. It's used to get a deep sample of your secretions), the team worried about my IVAD potentially being infected so they collected blood cultures from my IVAD port to ensure there wasn't anything brewing. This time when the team saw me and I explained my intensifying symptoms again and their reaction was different. Something made them worry about my piercing headaches being caused by meningitis. Once they said that I was officially scared. Transplant wipes out your immune system therefore your immunity, so all of my immunizations I've been getting since birth have all been wiped out.

I was advised to go to the emergency for further examination. We got to the emergency and I was terrified. At the time my neutrophil count was low therefore my immune system (ability to fight infections) was low. I was anxious about going into emergency and catching something but to my surprise after my mom wheeled me in on a wheelchair, they triaged me instantly, registered and in less than five minutes I was already being called into an assessment room. I felt like a mystery as physician after physician came into the room, asked 100 questions and left scratching their head. Post-transplant patients can be complex but just imagine a transplant patient with a pre-existing diagnosis of sickle cell disease. I was essentially a lab rat; I was that patient that everyone wanted to take a crack at so they could add it to their resumes. I was eventually admitted and taken to the Adult Hematology unit because they soon realized I was a complicated patient and this wasn't going to be quick. My eyes welled with tears the moment the nurse showed me to my room and walked away. This was the unit I spent so much time on pre-transplant and to be back on it after all of the stuff that I had just endured killed me. I started to question if it was all for nothing. My mind sped round and round wondering if these side effects meant my body was rejecting my sisters' cells. I still get emotional just remembering the pain I felt reliving one of my worst fears.

This hospital stay was a blur, I was constantly wheeled from test to test while the team tried to figure out what was going on. I had chest x-rays, ultrasounds, endless bloodwork and eventually the scariest part for me was the bronchoscopy which is essentially when you're taken to the operating room, semi sedated but still conscious, and your physician sticks a camera down your throat and explores. Yeah, doesn't sound too pleasant. They ended up finding that I had bacteria in my lungs that had caused an infection and likely some of my weird symptoms but it didn't seem to fully complete the puzzle. The team wanted to discharge me but with such low oxygen saturations it wasn't possible. I was kept for a few extra days then it occurred to a new set of eyes that maybe we should do a venous blood gas, which shows the level of gases in your blood. There it was right on the blood gas I had an unusual amount of methemoglobin, trust me even as a nurse I swear it was the first time I've ever heard of this. So methemoglobinemia was my official diagnosis which is a fancy way of saying I had lots of methemoglobin in my blood. This type of hemoglobin can carry oxygen but it doesn't drop it off to the tissues that need it.

Let's review the classic signs of methemoglobinemia: headache, shortness of breath, nausea, rapid heart rate, fatigue, confusion, and eventually loss of consciousness. So can someone tell me how this was missed since I was experiencing most of these symptoms. I was even told by the hematologist on ward that had I waited any longer to come to the hospital I could have had such little oxygen in my body and lost consciousness. As excited, I was that I finally had a diagnosis I was furious that I was initially told this was all due to my stress and anxiety. They concluded that this was caused by one of my antibiotics called Dapsone. I was put on this medication because of my allergy to penicillin and reaction to another antibiotic.

So essentially this was a medication reaction. Yes, my transplant pharmacist was in the room as I was reviewing my symptoms. I'm sure you can read my frustration. Honestly, I am a health professional so I 100% understand that people make mistakes and miss things, it comes with the job. My issue wasn't that something was missed, my issue was that when I saw the team again, they acted very nonchalant and didn't even apologize for what they previously told me. They didn't take any ownership for that fact that I was sitting in a hospital bed with real issues that a bubble bath and massage wasn't going to fix. So, after that encounter I made the decision that I wanted to be taken care of by a team that I felt supported and cared for. This decision didn't come easy and I am down playing all of the other drama that was associated with this. I am not a fan of the idea that a patient with an opinion is deemed a difficult patient. I believe my persistence was not well received and my knowledge of the system and how things worked became a barrier to forming a lasting relationship with this team. I would rather be deemed annoying, difficult and persistent if it meant that when it came time, I would save my life. That sounds dramatic but really it isn't. I honestly believe that if I didn't continue to harass and persist with my team to take me seriously, I would have stayed at home until I eventually went unconscious in the bathtub.

Please take my experience as a warning for your own life. Whatever situation you might be in health wise. You know yourself better than any book will tell a doctor about what you're experiencing. Listen to your body, if you think something is wrong and no one else is listening to you keep pushing. If they don't hear your voice, make it heard. Trust me you'll thank yourself later.

Bump Number Two: First Period Post-Transplant

Bump in the road two showed up about six months post-transplant. By now we all know that transplant conditioning can have an effect on your fertility. So, a major thing that was on my mind was when I would get my period again. My period stopped instantly after transplant and I was told getting it back would indicate that my body is beginning to wake up again. Well, it woke right up. It went from 0 to 100. When I saw that I finally got it, I was so excited! It meant that I was that much closer to getting better and hopefully to having a family of my own one day. I will spare you all the graphics but just know that I started bleeding and 21 days later I hadn't stopped. At this point I was worried. I called my transplant team and they were able to get me an emergency appointment with the fertility doctor I saw in Edmonton prior to freezing my eggs. I was immediately started on progesterone pills that should stop the bleeding and once under control I would start the nuva ring. The nuva ring is a type of birth control but in my case, it wasn't being used as contraception but rather hormone/period regulation. Usually, you put it in vaginally and leave it for 30 days then take it out for five to seven days and you get your period during that time. However, I was instructed to replace the old ring with a new one right away so I skipped my period entirely. I was losing so much blood and my blood counts had finally recovered so we didn't want to risk anything. It was nice to know that I had gotten my period but at the same time didn't have to deal with the weeks of bleeding anymore. Unfortunately, I still had to deal with the cramps but it's okay you win some you lose some.

Everything seemed to be looking up? Almost every problem had a solution, all asides from this one. During this fertility appointment I was given a full fertility work up and asked to come back in a week or so to review the results as well as the effectiveness of the progesterone. All of my fertility levels were checked (estradiol, luteinizing hormone, anti-mullerian hormone, prolactin, follicle stimulating hormone). I looked forward to hearing these results because if I already got my period and they weren't anticipating it would come back so fast it must mean that my body is doing a good job! I left that appointment devastated. Six months post-transplant I am sitting in a room with my fertility doctor and he is telling me that I should hurry up and have kids before my body goes into premature ovarian failure. After all that I felt like I was being left with a narrow window to have kids. He also mentioned that I couldn't even start trying for a child until six months after I am off my anti-rejections. I was on them for another six months and then six more months of recovery leaving me with what felt like a tiny window to potentially have children. I fought back tears and tried to be strong while he reassured me that I shouldn't stress about this. He continued telling me to enjoy my youth and don't jump into marriage and have kids too soon since I am now finally getting to live life. His encouraging words did the opposite, it reminded me that I was robbed of a life up until transplant and now felt like I was being robbed of a future. I walked through the hospital and back to my car in tears. Trying so hard to keep it together.

The moment I sat in my car I immediately erupted in tears. I was crying uncontrollably. I thought I covered all of my bases pre-transplant and knew exactly what I was getting myself into but man I was wrong. I called my sister and I could barely even speak between me catching my breath and crying. She was so worried and was ready to jump in her car to come and meet me in the parking lot so I didn't have to drive home. You know I'm always trying to be strong. I refused the help because I just wanted to drive home in silence then go straight to my room and forget this day ever happened. I could barely even tell my mom what I found out when I got home. I was a mess. My whole family was so worried. Then the thought that flooded my mind while I was in Calgary was back. "Was this even worth it" yes, six months post-transplant and I was still questioning if it was worth it. A large part of me regretted bringing all of these extra complications into my life because it didn't seem as if things were turning out how I had envisioned. The next few weeks I struggled with the idea that I was robbed of a lot of the joys of childhood, teenage years and young adulthood because of sickle cell disease. Now I had a transplant that was supposed to give me a new lease on life and I just found out that there might be a very short window of time I could have kids.

You better believe the next time I was down in Calgary for my monthly check up I furiously reviewed what my fertility doctor told me versus what I was told by the radiation specialist before transplant. My team had no answers for me other than "Revée, remember you are the first of this kind of transplant that we are doing so we knew going into this nothing was definite". They told me the poor results were likely due to the fact that fertility testing usually isn't completed until after one year when your body has had more time to heal. So, I calmed down and held unto the hope that maybe the testing was just done too early. This thought was enough to keep me from crying day in and day out but it wasn't enough to stop me from dwelling, stewing and pondering. But I made the decision that I was going to try and continue my life without this dark cloud hanging over me, it took a while to get there and honestly all of this fertility stuff still weighs down on me. I made the decision to trust that God has a plan for my life so I will continue to move forward and watch it come to fruition.

Bump Number Three: Iron Deficiency Anemia

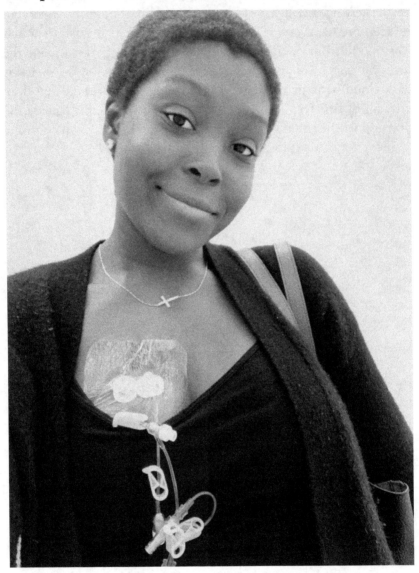

Not only is having a heavy period for three weeks annoying and uncomfortable, it also can have negative effects on your body. I was thrilled that I no longer had this ongoing period, but shortly after I began to feel weak, dizzy, light headed and fatigued. I was terrified that this was part two of my medication reaction. I told my doctor and I was brought in for more blood work and testing. Then there it was loud and clear in the blood work. I had an iron deficiency. At this point I was over this whole transplant recovery thing. I was beginning to feel like it was just one thing after another and that I couldn't catch a break. For two-three weeks at a time, I tried various iron pills to see which one worked and would drive my iron back up to a normal range. The first one wasn't so bad, didn't have any side effects from it but also when my blood work was done again it was clear that it wasn't working. So, I was changed to another one that was a bit stronger and had a different composition. It helped get my iron up slightly but man it killed my stomach. It felt like something was constantly gnawing at my stomach all hours of the day. I was struggling to eat and even function the pain was so bad. When I told my doctor about this, they realized that the impact of the medication was not worth the little bit that it made my iron increase. On to the next one, my doctor suggested iron infusions as a last resort. I was no stranger to infusions so I thought that it would be such a quick and easy thing. By now you should realize that most things don't come easy.

I went for my first iron infusion excited that I was five appointments away from feeling better. Five appointments until the dizziness, weakness, and fatigue was a thing of the past. I've had so many infusions over the years so I figured this would be a quick and easy in and out. I got to the unit, was prepped, IV initiated and hooked up. The infusion was dark brown and I watched my IV tubing slowly turn brown and the infusion into my vein. About five-ten minutes into the infusion I started feeling a bit of burning sensation at the injection site, I told the nurse and she told me not to worry it could just be my body getting used to the infusion. So, I decided to stand down and give it another five minutes. But then the pain intensified. Being a nurse myself I felt like something was wrong so I called the nurse again. She took a look at my arm again and it was now evident that my IV had gone interstitial aka meaning it was leaking out of the vein and under my skin. The infusion was slowed down and eventually stopped. My arm felt like it was on fire. The nurses figured that because they had such trouble getting the IV in, they may have punctured the vein causing the leak.

Try number two. This time I made sure that when the IV was being initiated, there was no fishing (that's the back-and-forth movement of the needle as the nurse tries to get blood flow back into the IV). The IV was gotten in one shot and the infusion started again. This time 15 minutes into the infusion my arm began to feel itching and my arm filled with tiny little bumps. I called the nurse over and it turns out yours truly was having a transfusion reaction to the iron. The infusion was stopped, the doctor was called and antihistamines were pushed immediately as they weren't sure how bad this reaction was going to be. Thankfully I had someone come with me so I didn't have to worry about driving home, since I was now partially sedated. They slowly infused the rest of the iron. On my way home I looked at the shadows on my arms, revealing bruises from IVs and tiny little bumps. I am not sure why but that was my turning point. My eyes filled with tears. I felt exhausted. I was beginning to feel like nothing would ever be easy or straightforward for me. Why couldn't one thing just go right? If having an iron deficiency wasn't bad enough, why couldn't the treatments come complication free? Frustrated but determined to get through this I powered through the next three iron infusions. The doctor now ordered for me to have pre-medications that would combat the reaction so I needed a driver every time because I knew I would be sedated. After about a month and a half of infusions I finally finished them and slowly began to feel better. My levels were rechecked and my iron was back within the normal range. So just like everything else there was another hurdle that I pushed through. It wasn't easy but I made it. This August took me back to my time in Calgary when I felt alone and isolated, but I will dive further into that a little bit later.

The take home message here again is that transplant comes with obstacles and as annoying or frustrating as they are you just have to push yourself through. Every issue has a solution but that doesn't mean that solution will come easily.

Bump Number Four: Unexplained Stomach Pains

We all know the saying "when it rains it pours". I was experiencing a case of one thing leading to another but thankfully this was the end of the line. It started with a period that wouldn't end, that led me to iron deficiency secondary to excessive blood loss that led us here. Stomach pain. As I discussed before, I started trialing various iron pills to find one that eventually worked. For anyone that's ever-taken iron pills before knows that they are HARD on the stomach. Add in trialing three different iron supplements with the other ten medications I was taking daily equals a very unhappy stomach. There is honestly nothing worse than a stomach ache that won't quit. The pain was so bad that it would wake me up in the middle of the night and I couldn't get back to bed. Leaving me exhausted the following day. There is really nothing worse than not having enough sleep. When you feel sleep deprived once or twice a week you usually can make it up later in the week. That wasn't quite the case for me because the pain was ongoing, a daily occurrence and so severe. I started taking a look at my diet to see if maybe there was a correlation between what I was eating and the pain. It seems even on the days I ate little to no oils, grease or fats and just stuck to veggies I was still woken up in the middle of the night in excruciating pain. No pain medication could control it, no amount of peppermint teas could soothe, and no number of Tums could settle my stomach.

One night the pain became so bad and was radiating to my back and my chest. I told my parents and they took me to the emergency. I spent the entire night with doctor after doctor coming in and out of my room asking the same questions and confused as to what could be going on. Sound Familiar? Regardless if I was pre- or post-transplant, I am still a mystery. X-rays were taken and ultrasounds performed. The only thing that the physicians saw was some inflammation in my stomach but with an unknown cause. On the bright side at least, I knew there was something really going on that was causing the pain and it wasn't in my head. I still had PTSD from the last time I brought issues forth. After discussing with my transplant team, the emergency room physicians pondered on the idea of my pain potentially being caused by GVHD. Yes, they said it, the words that I was afraid would eventually come out. I was told they would schedule for a scope so that they could go into my stomach via my rectum and cut a few specimens to analyze. Sounds pleasant right? Once the pain was under control I was discharged from the hospital, then a few days later I was at the pharmacy collecting a giant jug of Colyte. I was given specific instructions from the pharmacist regarding how much of the solution you had to drink and when you had to drink it. So Colyte was a powdered solution that you add 2L of water to and it becomes your gastro prep, meaning it's going to clear everything out of your system so when the camera is inserted the physician can have a good look. I won't lie, the prep night was a hard night, it gets to the point when you've cleared out so much that your stomach is empty but you still have the urge to run to the washroom. Oh man, I honestly wouldn't wish that on my worst enemy. Anyways I survived the evening/night that led into D-Day. I still had half of the solution to drink the morning of. I really wondered what the point of that was, I swear my system was already wiped clean. I made my way to the hospital with my mom as the driver and we showed up at the endoscopy unit, briefly waited in a room full of people and then I was called in. I went to the bathroom and changed into the gown, I nervously looked at myself gowned up in the mirror and just began to pray that whatever was going on was anything but GVHD. Laid back down on the stretcher, an IV was started and I was wheeled in the procedure room. The anesthesiologist began pushing medications and placed oxygen on me. I closed my eyes because I was terrified of this conscious sedation idea. I closed my eyes and woke up. Who knows how long later and caught a glimpse of my insides up on the big screen but immediately fell back asleep. Once the procedure was over the doctors came out of the room and told me that they are in the process of analyzing the specimens they collected but thus far it wasn't looking like GVHD. I could finally breathe again. In the end it was found that my stomach lining had just become damaged from all of the medications I have been on in the last year and it seemed like the iron pills were the tipping point that pushed my stomach over the edge. Essentially my stomach was functioning in a constant state of inflammation so I was advised to try and combat that inflammation by cutting out foods that cause inflammation. Sounds easy enough, right? Wrong everything causes inflammation it seemed.

What's A FODMAP?

I started on something called the low FODMAP diet. You're probably wondering what the heck that is? Trust me I was wondering the same thing. So FODMAP is an acronym for fructans, oligosaccharides, disaccharides, monosaccharides and polyols. I know you're still wondering what that is. So those are short chain carbohydrates and sugars that are not well absorbed in the body and can lead to stomach pain and bloating. These were adding to my horrible stomach pain. A lot of different foods fall under this category and a lot of fruits and vegetables, so the days when I thought I was eating healthy to make my stomach feel better I was actually doing the opposite. Two of my favourite foods that I had to cut out were onion and garlic. You might think that's not too bad but in every African dish lies onion and garlic as well as any canned marinade or sauce. So, I was on that plain salt and pepper diet. I also cut out dairy and gluten so in reality I wasn't left with anything tasty. I thought I was going to starve to death. I downloaded a low FODMAP app that allows you to look up different foods and it will let you know if it was high, medium or low in FODMAPs. Most of the time I was discouraged and so upset because it felt like everything was high risk. I cried sometimes when I opened the fridge and saw so many tasty things my family were enjoying but I couldn't. I thank God for my mom making special low FODMAP versions of my favourite African dishes. My boyfriend at the time constantly found ways to make me feel better about my meal plan. One day he showed up at my place with a big bag of groceries so we could make a healthy low FODMAP friendly date night meal. It was the little things like that which made me feel like things were going to get better. Hanging out with my friends became harder and harder because literally everything we do surrounds food. I don't know if it's the same for you or if maybe my friends and I are foodies. Going to the mall meant shopping then having lunch, going for coffee also meant getting a fast-food snack, going for a walk meant stopping for a slurpee too. It was tough but once my friends realized the situation, we found ways to still get together and either incorporate low FODMAP foods or no food at all.

After I realized, I wasn't going to die of starvation this whole low FODMAP thing wasn't so bad. It actually gave me an opportunity to bust out of my tiny food comfort zone and experiment with new recipes. I actually began enjoying making different kinds of foods and testing out different low FODMAP spices. I also saved a lot of money because I wasn't really able to eat out, knowing that most fast foods are packed with FODMAPs. I forced myself to plan my meals ahead of time and prep snacks that I could take along with me. I explored different stores in Edmonton that sold gluten free/ lactose free options. I tried my best to make the best of a difficult situation and it made me more mindful of the things I was putting in my mouth and it birthed a new love for taking care of my body. We all are given situations that suck, but are you trying your best to find the silver lining? As bad as it was, at least I lost weight, right? Haha take a second and think about whatever you're dealing with and find your silver lining.

CHAPTER TWENTY-SIX

MIND OVER MATTER

For the most part I was excellent at finding silver linings. I was truly known as the person who wore rose coloured glasses. I saw life with so much optimism and positivity for the most part and I really believe that mindset is what carried me through my sickle struggles and eventually transplant. So, what happened next was shocking to me. What do you do when you break or lose your rose-colored glasses? And life now looks gloomy? Honestly, I didn't know what to do and that's why it became a problem. About five-six months post-transplant I fell into a depression that I didn't think I'd be able to find my way out. It's funny because in Calgary the psychologist I saw during transplant warned me about this potentially happening. At the time I didn't really believe I belonged to that statistic. But when the sadness hit it HIT. It was mostly a combination of things that I've already mentioned in the book thus far but let's break it down.

Expectation Vs. Reality

It started with the classic expectation versus reality. This was my own mistake, I believed that transplant would make my life easier, not only would I be cured but my life would be easier in general. I figured that the majority of my struggles all stemmed from sickle cell disease. Which was true to some degree. But once I became sickle cell free, I was still dealing with the ongoing and what felt like never ending side effects of transplant. The hospital visits just reminded me so vividly of what I was trying to get away from. The fatigue that I experienced honestly lasted all through my first-year post-transplant. It was so discouraging to be excited to experience this new life but then feel the weight of all the restrictions. I still had to be careful of where I went because I was still on immune suppressants. My diet was still restricted due to still being immuno-compromised. The news about my fertility really made me spiral. It was the one thing that had the potential to hold me back from going through with a transplant in the first place. I was devastated. I truly believed that my future had been taken away. I felt like I was robbed of so many experiences growing up due to sickle cells and now to feel like even though I am cured I am still going to miss out on things I want most in the future. I just wanted something in my life to be easy and to be straight forward.

Comparison

Another thing was comparison. Comparison really is the thief of joy. I spent so much time looking right and left at all of the beautiful things my friends were doing and accomplishing. I am the type of person that allows my friends' successes to motivate me to do better, I always celebrate other people's wins because I knew my win was coming. But when my rose coloured glasses broke. I found it so hard to believe that there was anything good coming for me. I began to believe that my life was just going to be a series of unfortunate events. At the time I had a boyfriend and the summer after transplant we hit our three-year anniversary, for any 20–30-year-old woman. By three years you begin to expect a bit of progression in your relationship, in terms of either engagement or living together. I didn't believe in living with anyone until engagement and my partner knew that. I felt like transplant not only put my life on hold but really my relationship on hold as well. During my time in Calgary, we spent so much time planning our future together and the only hurdle it seemed we had to overcome was getting out of the hospital and getting healthy. So, when I got back to Edmonton, I figured that my relationship would just fall into place, he'd propose and by one-year post-transplant we would be planning our wedding. Obviously, I was wrong because I am currently single and not engaged as I write this. What I didn't realize at the time was that transplant really does take a toll on the people that are close to you. I figured my mom would be the only one really affected because she had to uproot her life and physically be in Calgary with me. I was wrong, my entire family struggled in some way and my partner as well. The mental strain of transplant seemed to take a toll on him and he didn't quite feel ready to progress our relationship to marriage. My dreams of this perfect life post-transplant were crushed. I figured since he was patient and so supportive towards me during transplant that I owed him the same respect of giving him time to figure things out. We eventually broke up just before our fourth-year anniversary. But life goes on and I couldn't be more thankful that I had his support during my darkest days.

My Community

Losing what I thought was my identity. Have you ever had a job that you loved so much and it pretty much became your world? Before you know it, you start telling everyone that's where you work before they even ask and then slowly but surely it becomes "you." That's kind of what happened to me. I worked in the neonatal intensive care unit (NICU) since I had my final nursing preceptorship. The area sparked my interest because my niece was born at 25 weeks and spent three months there. That experience really opened my eyes to the world of intensive care nursing. So, I set my sights on it and before I knew it, I landed my first job out of nursing school there. I loved the babies, the responsibility, the autonomy and the challenge this unit brought to my life. It helped me develop my skills as a new nurse and it began to become a part of my identity. I felt proud to work there and even prouder to play such a big role in these families lives. Due to my sickle cells progressing I had to drop down to part time and then eventually leave the unit for a lower intensity clinic job. Then took medical leave for the duration of transplant and recovery. I felt detached from my old coworkers, and from my skill set. The same feeling bled into my friendships. I began to feel like I didn't quite fit in with them as we were in such different stages of our lives. Because I was beginning to lose my positivity, I realized that I no longer was that motivating and inspiring friend. I felt like the Debby downer friend and the thought of being that person just drove me further and further away from the people I cared about. And of course, once you go down that rabbit hole good luck trying to get out. I know it's crazy but when you're down you're down.

Surprisingly enough even being cured from sickle cells actually took some adjustment for me. Imagine your whole life you're known for something whether it's where you live, work, or something you may possess, when it's gone it takes time to adjust to your new normal. I was surprised by this because I knew that going through transplant would potentially make me sickle cell free but I never really understood what it meant to be sickle cell free. Although it was a great thing, it was the highest form of blessing and miracle I could ever imagine, but it still was hard for me. I no longer fit into the sickle cell community because now I was "cured". The bond that I had formed with other patients with sickle cell all of a sudden didn't feel the same. They looked at me like the "lucky one" that made it to the other side. We used to be able to talk about how we managed our pain crises and the struggles that life with sickle cell disease brought us. Now all of a sudden, I was put into a position where I no longer could relate to their pain because as they were describing their current pain and I was talking about the past.

Not only did I struggle to fit in with the sickle cell community, I also struggled to fit into the transplant population either. I felt like the odd man out, submerged into a cancer world but still on the outside. Have you ever felt like an outsider? I promise, no one ever said anything to me saying that I didn't belong but it's not always what people say but it's how they act. Sometimes I did feel that when medical professionals saw the type of chemotherapy I had and the dose of radiation on my file they almost scoffed at it. Often it was insinuated that my treatment was "easy" as opposed to what they have seen before. Which is fair enough, maybe they have seen much heavier and scarier treatment but this was my experience. Also, I was taking a chance and risked being the first person in my province or maybe even country to embark on this journey, so I thought I deserved a bit of credit. There is an outpouring of support and funding available for cancer patients but the sickle cell patient that had the cancer like treatment wasn't able to partake in most of them. It was similar to the general population I was too sick to relate to but then in the cancer world oftentimes I felt like I was not sick enough. This made it so hard to feel comfortable in any space. This continued to feed into my idea that no one really understood what I was going through. I was trying my best to stay afloat and manage all of the disappointments and discouragements but this next one set me over the edge. The combination of everything I already discussed with this news on top of it, I was ready to throw in the towel.

CHAPTER TWENTY-SEVEN

PATIENT TURNED CAREGIVER

As I mentioned earlier my mom was my caregiver and physically had to pack her belongings up and move to Calgary with me. So, when we came back to Edmonton just as I had so many follow up appointments, she also needed to catch up on four months of her own appointments. As every woman over 50 is expected to do, my mom had to get her mammogram. Before getting the results, our family doctor noticed some "speckles" on the images but she reassured us that it was likely just calcium build up and nothing to worry about but when the official results were in, she would call us. Once the results were in, she called my mom for an appointment, I decided to go with her to that appointment because the crazy in me needed to get a copy of the official report that showed it was just calcium build up. We got to the office and waited for the doctor. She entered the room with a look on her face that didn't look like someone who was about to tell us that it was nothing. She started explaining that these speckles were not calcium and actually looked like cancer cells. She went on to say "I'm so sorry Margaret you have cancer" at that point I am pretty sure I blacked out.

I looked at my mom being the strong black woman that she always is, staring straight at the doctor and trying to take it in. I could feel my body get hot and my eyes begin to swell with tears. The doctor reassured us that my mom is very lucky because we caught it so early that with intervention, she'd beat this thing in no time. The doctor continually apologized and then gave me the official report that I was hoping for but unfortunately the report didn't say what I had hoped. I gave my mom a big hug and told her it was going to be okay and we would get through this. At the time I don't even remember if I believed that but I knew I needed to support and motivate my mom the same way she did for me. We got into the car and called my dad, when he answered he sounded so eager to hear that this was all nothing and just a scare. My mom couldn't even speak at this point she was so upset. The only words I could get out were "mom has cancer" that was all he needed to know. Just saying the C word made my eyes fill with tears. We called my siblings and told them the news. The entire family was in shock and disbelief. I drove us home and went straight to my room when we got home, at this point I was a mess. I felt like I was living in a nightmare.

My whole family met up that evening in my parents living room. All staring at the official document like the harder we looked we would find an error. Unfortunately, that didn't happen. We spent that evening combing through all of the details of this diagnosis and doing some research into different options. Even though we all knew she was being referred to a specialist and someone would guide us through this process, we loved being prepared and well informed. In between the conversation we all looked at each other in silence, even though no one was saying anything it was pretty clear that we all felt like there was no way our family was dealing with another major health event. It really felt unfair. I couldn't wrap my head around the idea that the person who took care of me at my worst was being repaid with a cancer diagnosis once we finally thought life was about to get better. Our one saving grace at this time was that because we saw what God did for me, we were reassured that He could do it for my mom.

My mom embarked on this journey with unshakable faith, and confidence that was almost annoying. At the time there was a part of me that really wanted her to just be upset and angry about this diagnosis. Honestly, I felt like I was more upset, scared and angry about it than she was. Now I realize she was really just channeling the healing testimony that God gave me to motivate her through her own health journey. We often forget the blessings of testimonies. I watched my mom cruise through this experience with poise, confidence and faith. From every oncologist appointment, to surgery consultation, to radiation treatment, to follow up support groups, to physiotherapy appointments, to exercise programs to help her regain her strength, my mom powered through as if she already knew that God was going to heal her. During this journey my mom underwent a lumpectomy surgery in May, followed by 16 rounds of radiation to her chest and breast in August. It was a really tough time for my mom and for the entire family. It felt like the roles were reversed and it was my turn to pay it forward. I still wasn't fully recovered and simultaneously I was dealing with a 21-day period, disappointing fertility news, iron deficiency, trialing multiple pills, and eventually iron infusions. I thank God for giving me the strength to endure all of this because trust me there were days where I was about to crumble. I just couldn't believe my mom and I were going through so much at once. There were days that I would drive my mom to the Cancer Institute in the morning, wait for her to complete radiation, we'd go home and rest, then in the afternoon she would be driving me to the University Hospital to get my iron infusions. In the end after all of my mom's interventions she was healed, and cancer free! We praise God! With God as her protector, we already know she will remain cancer free!

CHAPTER TWENTY-EIGHT

MENTAL HEALTH

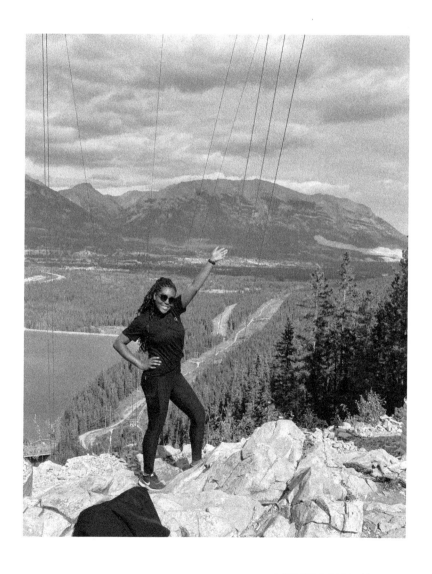

Now you have a better understanding as to why my mental health was really struggling during this time, let's talk about how I got out of this dark headspace. When they say you have to put the work in for the outcomes you want, the same goes for mental health. I was sent to a psychologist when I returned to Edmonton that was helping me adjust to my new life back home. I would check in with her on a monthly basis and as time progressed, she started to notice some changes in my thought patterns, the way I saw life and my emotions. She told me she believed I was depressed and she wanted to refer me to a psychiatrist to chat with me about the potential for medication. Hearing that I was shocked. I knew I was sad at times and I always carried a level of anxiety but this was different. It took me a while to even accept that I was experiencing depression. On my way home from that appointment, I called my sister and told her what the psychologist had said and she was just as shocked as I was. She encouraged me that I had to share this with my parents so they understood what I was going through. For anyone that grew up in a very Christian or Catholic African home you can probably relate to anxiety I was having about sharing this with my parents. My parents are lovely, however mental health issues were not something that they grew up learning and talking about. Like most people we put value on physical illness because you can see it but mental health you can't. I vividly remember the day I told my parents that I was feeling depressed. They were shocked and then the first thing that my dad said was "What do you have to be depressed about?" My parents were legitimately confused because they understood why I would have been depressed before transplant when I was told there was no cure. But now that I have been cured of this horrible disease, how could I be upset or even depressed. I felt guilty that I had essentially gotten what I wanted but I still was unhappy. The guilt fed into the depression I was already feeling and made it worse. My thoughts all became negative and the silver lining I used to search for was long gone. At this point I knew I needed help.

Recovery

Here are a few things that I did that worked for me. They might not help everyone but they definitely helped me. I understand that everyone has access to different services so I urge you to look into your community and see what services you can access if you're ever struggling. Before you can even get started with recovery you need to acknowledge how you're feeling. Be honest with yourself and come to terms with the fact that you are feeling down. Be kind to yourself. Remind yourself that no one is perfect and everyone is allowed to have down days.

Seek Help

Talk to someone you can trust. Whether that person is a family member, friend, pastor or peer. Sometimes just saying how you feel out loud can provide a sense of relief. I was already seeing a psychologist but I increased my visits with her to every two weeks, then decided to have check ins with the psychologist I was with before transplant every two months and lastly saw a psychiatrist monthly. Talk about putting the work in! At the time it didn't really feel like any of these things were helping me but it seems the combination of all helped in the end. I was never started on any antidepressants, we found that a large contributor to the way I was feeling was actually lack of sleep. My stomach issues I mentioned before were keeping me up late and waking me up in the middle of the night leading to exhaustion. When it happens once or twice you can usually bounce back but because it was constant it began to get to me. We trialed so many different sleeping pills and, in the end, what helped was melatonin and a sleep meditation app.

Join A Support Group

I know it sounds geeky but it honestly helped me a lot. I attended two support groups. One was YAC which was young adult's cancer support, I didn't have cancer but I fell into that category because of the treatments I received. This group was run out of a volunteer run cancer facility, we would meet weekly to play games, chat and have snacks. I liked this group because it was like this unspoken thing that we have all be through some traumatic health events and some were still in the midst of theirs. We didn't have to talk about what we were going through but there was an understanding that you couldn't get elsewhere. It was nice to lay down your worries at the door when you entered the facility then just have fun and connect with people with similar experiences.

The second group I went to was biweekly. It was run though the cancer hospitals psychology department. Every session had a different discussion topic that was let by a social worker or a psychologist. It was an opportunity to share your story and hear other people's stories. It was nice to hear that even though no one had the same journey as me we all could relate on how our experiences with health and treatments have impacted our lives. Honestly it was the first time in a while I felt like I belonged somewhere. People that understood the fear I felt laying on the radiation bed as well as experiencing post-chemo side effects. We all had different journeys but we could come together and relate. These sessions often resulted in tears, hugs and feelings of belonging and joy. I am so thankful I had the opportunity to participate in these sessions.

Get Outside & Start Walking

I loved getting outside for a walk, not only because I was trying to build my endurance but in was nice to go out and enjoy nature. Sometimes I'd go for a walk with a friend but other times I would put some praise and worship music on and walk on my own. It was a time to think and talk to God. I probably was deemed that weirdo on the path that was constantly talking or singing to herself. I always returned home with a clear head and a smile on my face.

Exercise

I joined the ACE program (Alberta Cancer Exercise) which was a rehabilitation exercise program that provided guided exercise three times a week. It was tailored to you in terms of your fitness level, skill level and stage in treatment. You work with a group of people all different ages, sexes and types of cancers. Again, as I mentioned before I just fell into the cancer world. When I started the program, I could barely even do one sit up, hold myself up above the ground to do a plank or even walk for ten minutes without becoming exhausted. The trainers worked with me multiple times a week, pushed me in ways I never would be able to push myself and motivated me to keep at it even when I was ready to give up. By the end of this 12-week program I could hold a plank for over one minute when previously I couldn't even hold my body up. It doesn't sound like that much but to me it was a big deal. I set the goal that I wanted to learn how to run so eventually I could enter a 5k run. I am still working on running and I still hope to run 5k one day. Setting fitness goals for myself really helped me focus on something that I could finally control. During this recovery there were so many things that I wasn't able to control but this I could work at and see results. Made me feel like I was in control again.

Continue Doing The Things You Love & Brings You Joy

Sometimes when you feel down the first response is to completely disengage with things around you. I found that the further away you feel from your "normal" the worse you feel. I forced myself to continue journaling, connecting with family, and laughing as much as I could.

Learn Something New or Master An Old Skill

My mom and I took up knitting to help up pass the time. I knew how to knit before but I was never super confident in it. All this free time gave me the opportunity to try my hand at strengthening that skill. Before I knew it, I was teaching my mom and we were knitting scarfs for my entire family. It was nice to feel accomplished at something because I didn't really feel like I was accomplishing anything.

Surround Yourself With People That Uplift You

This might be one of the things that helped me the most. Have you ever hung out with a friend and on the way home you are thinking "wow they are just so amazing" that friend that leaves you feeling full of positivity? These are the type of people you want to surround yourself with when times are tough, they will encourage you, inspire you and continually motivate you. You do not want to surround yourself with people that will suck the energy out of you when you are already running on empty. Sometimes we don't realize what an impact the people around us have on our mental health but I urge you to be mindful and choose the right support system to help you through. That support system might be big or small, maybe made up of immediate or extended family, perhaps school or work friends but whoever you choose to surround yourself with ensure their presence fills you up not brings you down.

Hold On To Something Positive

Whether that is a positive memory, a goal you hope to achieve or a milestone you are working towards, try not to lose sight of it. My something positive was knowing that my nieces and nephews loved me dearly and needed me around. I would reminisce on the fun activities we used to do together and remind myself that I just need to get better so we could make more memories together.

Spend Time Developing Your Spirituality

Last but definitely not least. If you are a Christian spend time with God. My spiritual and devotional life grew exponentially during this recovery period. The more time I spent with God the less time I had to dwell and ruminate on the tough stuff. God provided me with a comfort and ease that nothing/ no-one else could. The more I read my bible the closer I felt to God and the smaller I felt my problems were. If you've never believed in a higher power before and you're going through some tough stuff, this might be the perfect time to incorporate something new into your life.

It definitely took me a while and a lot of work but in the end, God was able to pull me out of the darkest place I have ever been. And if you're currently in that same place I was, I pray God will deliver you from that terrifying place. But remember, yes God will save you but you also have to put the work in to get better. It wasn't easy but I am so happy to be on the other side. When I look back, I honestly wonder how I could have felt so down when there were so many blessings around me that I just couldn't see. It's hard when your rose coloured glasses break or get lost but I thank God that I found mine again because my life is much brighter with them on.

CHAPTER TWENTY-NINE

MY NEW NORMAL

Acceptance

It took me a while but I was finally at a place of acceptance. I accepted that I had sickle cell disease, I accepted that I had a stem cell transplant to cure it, I accepted that due to this I might have challenges having children, I accepted that this process was extremely traumatic, I accepted that this was an opportunity to grow, I accepted that I am a new person because of this experience, I accepted that this experience made me unique, I accepted that I was now on a journey to find my new normal and most of all I accepted that this was God's plan for my life and I am exactly where He intended for me to be. The moment I began to accept that this was the life that I was given the more I began to see my situation as a blessing rather than a burden. I realized that sickle cells and transplant was not a curse but an opportunity for God to show his strength, power and might. There is really and truly no testimony without a test. God takes our toughest situations and turns them into something beyond on wildest dreams.

I learned to be patient with my body and allow myself the time and space I needed to recover. Instead of rushing the process I was leaning into the process and enjoying every moment of it. I was given a chance to write a new script for my story, there were so many barriers and restrictions placed on my life with sickle cells. All of a sudden, those barriers were removed and I was handed a blank canvas. I was almost overwhelmed with all of the freedom and opportunity that laid in front of me. I began exploring some things that I was told I couldn't do because of my illness and finding ways to accomplish them. A big one for me was swimming, sickle cells made swimming such a terrifying experience because almost every time I set foot in a pool, I would end up in sickle cell crisis. The cold water made my vessels constrict making it easier for my sickled cells to get stuck and create blockages as they roamed my body. So, I fearfully took adult swimming lessons hoping that nothing would happen to me. I soon realized that my swimming aversion actually has turned into a fear of getting into a pool. I was so nervous on my first lesson, and was ready to walk out. But I forced myself to believe that my only barrier was my sickle cells and now that is gone, I had no excuse not to be able to swim. After months of weekly lessons, I actually learned how to swim, I can't say I am the best but I am definitely getting the hang of it. I mentioned earlier in the book that I had so many transplant related eating restrictions that made it hard to feel normal. As time progressed my restrictions lifted and it was fun to get back to eating foods that I wasn't able to. The first time I had soft serve ice cream or ordered sushi were such milestones. It made me stop looking at life from a perspective of being deprived to the excitement of re-trying old favourites and savouring each moment.

Another big step to my new normal life was the removal of my port. My port was used for my red cell exchange treatments after my femoral vessels became to scarred to use anymore. That gizmo saved me from so many failed IV attempts and painful line inser-tions into scarred vessels. As I mentioned before my port was bur-ied deep within my right breast tissue, low enough that it could be hidden under some clothes but high enough that it was accessible. My transplant and hematology teams figured it was best for me to keep it in until I was at least a year post-transplant just in case for any reason I needed it again. When I got the call that an OR was finally being set up, I was so excited, it was one more reassurance that I was getting better and moving further and further way from transplant. The removal surgery went well asides that fact that when I said it was a part of me, I wasn't joking, the surgeon was literally struggling to remove it. My skin had grown so tightly around it and really didn't want to part with me. Let me tell you that this surgery was done awake so I felt like I was being rocked side to side as the surgeon struggled. Eventually it was out and my chest felt empty. Every morning I would feel for it out of routine but every morning to my surprise it wasn't there. Often times I even forget I had a port at all. I might be wearing a lower cut shirt and someone would point at the line across my chest and ask me what that was from? Initially I would look at it like, "what are you talking about" then I'd look down and realize what they were referring to. I used to hate this scar but eventually I began to like that I had a built-in conversation starter and battle wound. Every time I look in the mirror this scar reminds me of what I've been through and how blessed I am to be where I am today.

Acceptance allowed me to really live each day feeling blessed and extremely grateful for the life I was given. I was given a second chance at life and I refused to waste it. I began viewing my body like a temple. I became more mindful of the foods that I put in my body as well as the medications. I spent my entire life reliant on medication to survive. People who knew me before transplant will be able to speak to the fact that I didn't go anywhere without a bag of painkillers with me. I would often take the medication even before I had pain, I thought I was taking it preventatively so that if for some reason pain was to come out of nowhere while I was out and about, I was already a step ahead. Popping Advil and Tylenol like they were candy and feeling no relief, so doubling the dose was my normal. Every hospital admission I was pumped with some type of IV pain medication and then injected with an anti-nausea every two-four hours. It was chemical after chemical to "stay healthy" and "feel better". I decided that I was going to try my hand at living a more natural lifestyle in terms of trying to eliminate excess chemicals. I took to the internet and began looking for natural homemade swaps for some of my favourite things. I spent hours on end learning about the benefits of different essential oils and how to incorporate them into my life. I began with natural body products for myself and my family because if I was getting healthy, I was going to encourage them to do the same. I made lip chaps, body butters, and deodorants. It was fun to experiment and come out with the perfect combinations. Shortly after I dived into the natural cleaning products world. The cleaning products stemmed from the fact that I would feel sick and light headed every time I would clean the bathroom. It was probably partially the chemicals circulating but also that sterile clean bleach scent reminded me too vividly of my days in the hospital. So, I worked hard to find alternatives. In the end I made kitchen cleaners, bathroom cleaners, glass cleaners and air fresheners. This quickly transitioned from a hobby to a lifestyle. I switched out all of my plug-in air fresheners for diffusers with essential oils. I disposed of my heavy-duty pain killers and replaced them with essential oil roller balls. The more I learned the more passionate I became about healthy living and the effects of some the products we expose ourselves to and environments we place ourselves in. I am so thankful transplant opened my eyes to the value of being mindful of the things I introduce into my life.

Business

After months of testing and trialing products, in September 2020 I launched a natural product line. My brand is called Rêve Naturals and my goal is to help individuals achieve their dream skin, hair and home the natural way. All of my products are handmade in small batches, low ingredient, cruelty free and of course packed with lots of love! I currently sell a light and fluffy whipped body butter, a smooth and creamy whipped hair butter, a minty fresh lip butter and lastly a sweet and spicy room mist. I thank God for the experiences that have led me to starting this business. If you're looking for healthier alternatives to your daily products, take some time to visit my website www.revenaturals.com.

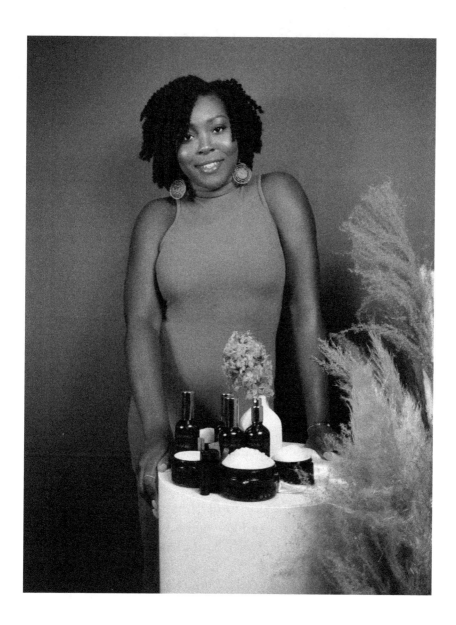

Finding Purpose

Once I fully accepted my experience, I was able to confidently step into the purpose that God had for my life. For a long time, I didn't believe that God had a purpose for me. I truly did believe that I was forgotten and maybe even here by accident. I didn't believe God had a plan for me this whole time but I just needed to step into it. I was given such a blessing and there was no way I couldn't share it with the world. Despite my fears and hesitations, I began sharing my testimony of healing on Instagram. I am a very private person so I was very hesitant to share my life so publicly because we all know once it's on the internet it's there for good. After leaving Calgary I told myself that I wanted to live my life paying it forward. All of the kindness and blessings that I had the privilege to experience, wasn't something that I could just keep locked up and throw away the key. I decided it was time to be open and honest. To my surprise the response was amazing. Friends, family and strangers began to follow my sickle cell advocacy page. This gave me momentum to continue making YouTube videos to find more ways to share my story. I spent my free time filming videos, editing videos, creating content and ultimately building a brand. I turned my empty days that made me question if I even wanted to get out of bed, to jumping out of bed every morning feeling like I had a purpose and was really impacting lives. I loved reading comments and hearing that the content I was putting out was lifting peoples' spirits. People felt inspired and motivated by hearing my story. I was shocked that my story was touching people to this extent. I am just little old me? A sick girl made well. It seemed that this idea of overcoming obstacles was something that so many people could relate to and not just those with sickle cells but anyone that ever experienced any type of health struggle. It felt amazing to inspire people and use my story to keep others going through hard times. Even when you feel like your life is boring or your story is nothing anything one would relate to, share it. You never know who needs to hear what you have to say. You never know who feels alone, stuck or hopeless and your story is exactly what they need.

I made inspiring people with my story my focus and before I knew it my transplant video that was filmed by Alberta Health Services was increasing in views daily, my sister and I were being interviewed on the news regarding our experience with transplant. I was featured in a medical journal, as well as our provincial health magazine. I was being interviewed on podcasts and asked to speak at conferences. I am so thankful that I have been given so many blessings and opportunities thus far in my life and I look forward to all the other amazing things God has in store for my future.

CHAPTER THIRTY

WALKING IN PURPOSE

After over a year of recovery, growth, and re-discovering myself I felt it was time for me to try and venture back into the workforce. My medical leave was extended until November which would be a full two years off but in March, I became more interested in seeing what kind of jobs were available that I could do. My physicians recommended that if I was going to head back to work, I should try and find something that was clinic based or wouldn't require me to do shift work and work nights as well as was part-time or could offer me a gradual return to work. So, I scoured our provincial website for opportunities that fit the bill. Eventually I found some and sent my resumes absolutely everywhere, after about a month I began to get a few call backs. I was excited but nervous that I had to find a way to turn my brain back on to prepare for these interviews. It might sound crazy but the nurse part of my brain had been turned off for so long that I wasn't really sure how I was supposed to turn it back on so quickly. Some of these interviews required a math exam, which coming from the NICU shouldn't have been a problem. But it was. I swear I couldn't remember how to do basic math and when I got the answer I would doubt and second guess myself. After lots of questions sent to previous coworkers to help me prepare for the math exams and interviews it was finally time.

In a three-week period of time, I went to five different interviews. Some were good and some were bad. The first one I had I was offered the job but unfortunately had to decline because they wouldn't be able to accommodate a gradual return to work. I was devastated because this job checked off all my boxes but I figured

I had many more interviews coming up so more opportunities. To my surprise, the four other jobs called me back and I was told I wasn't the successful applicant. As painful as it was, I took it as a sign that God was trying to tell me that I wasn't ready to go back to work. A few weeks later my sister mentioned to me that she heard of a position posting where I would be able to work with pediatric sickle cell patients. So, I went back online and did some searching, eventually there it was, the job of my dreams. The successful applicant would be a part of the pediatric hematology clinic and work directly with sickle cell disease patients. I wanted this job more than I have ever wanted any job. This job was the exact reason why I wanted to become a nurse in the first place. It was because of a sickle cell disease nurse that impacted me in so many ways. I wanted the opportunity to be the nurse that goes above and beyond for my patients and advocates for them in ways others couldn't. I applied and didn't hear anything for a week. My sister had a contact who was able to give me the name of the unit manager and one of the physicians I have met before that worked there. So, I reached out to them with my resume and cover letter, then a few days later I got a phone call for an interview. I researched everything I could about this position and made sure I knew the ins and outs of what my job would entail. The days following the interview were absolutely painful. I wanted this job so bad but at the same time I knew that my going back to work was in God's hands. Eventually I got a call back from the manager and she offered me the job only on the occasion that I could have all of my paperwork in order by the end of the week, giving me five days. That wouldn't be too hard if I wasn't just coming fresh off of medical leave. By paper work she meant I had to get my nursing license reinstated as it was currently non-practicing (this process generally takes three weeks), complete my fit to work assessment with my physician, have it submitted to HR so I can be officially taken off medical leave (which takes about two weeks to see my doctor for the assessment, then however long it takes for HR to process and deem me fit to work), sign up for CPR (which is only offered weekly and often is full months in advance) and get my N95 mask fit (which could be done with CPR). So naturally I was extremely discouraged because I felt like I was being asked to complete an impossible task. I said to the manager with confidence that I could get it done but in reality, I didn't believe that. This is where God stepped in. I called to get my nursing license changed to practicing and I was told that it takes a few weeks, I explained my situation but the lady said that she doesn't think getting it done in five days was possible. In three days, I got a call and it was completed, first item done. I called to book an appointment with my doctor that generally takes weeks. They had a spot available in an hour, so I got dressed and went immediately. My doctor filled out the necessary forms right in front of me and I was able to scan and sent to HR by the end of the day. My BMT team provided a fitness to work letter and that was also sent. I went online to book CPR and there randomly was a class coming up in three days, and there was room for one more. I completed CPR and got my mask fit done. I called my manager a day earlier than she expected to let her know I completed all of the tasks she asked. She was even shocked by how fast I was able to get everything done, she congratulated me and sent me the offer letter that evening. I officially got the job. Talking about this story brings tears to my eyes because again God made a way for me when there was clearly no apparent way. I started the job the following Monday. I immediately fell in love with my role and with the fact that I got to play such a big part in the lives of sickle cell patients.

"I am so happy to see that my sister is now healthy and doing well. It's surreal to see her accomplishing dreams that previously seemed out of reach" - Dimitri.

All of a sudden it made sense to me. Getting this job honestly put all of the puzzle pieces together. From the day I was born and eventually diagnosed with sickle cell disease God had a plan for my life. All of my hospital stays as a child were planned, the fact that I was alone and terrified in the hospital when my parents had to leave for the night and the nurse was the only one there to comfort me, eventually became the reason why I wanted to be a nurse in the first place. I wanted to make people feel like they were not alone, I wanted to hold their hand through their tough times and I wanted to be able to bring light into a dark situation. The fact that I was on Hydroxyurea and it failed me leading me to red cell exchange that eventually failed me as well was planned.

The thirst and desire I had to find a cure was all part of the plan. Now I am working in a position where I get to use my nursing knowledge as well as my past experiences to provide my patients with information, support, guidance and encouragement. I get to be the person that these children with sickle cells will look up to and realize that you can achieve greatness even with this disease. God used me to reveal His glory. At the time I really didn't see that, but getting this job just put everything in place. I am walking in the purpose that God put me on this planet for. There are often days when I am driving to work and I begin to cry because I am in awe of what God has done for me and the fact that I get the opportunity every single day to pay it forward leaves me speechless. You really never know what God has for you. If you would have told me at 12 when I first researched sickle cells that I would be in this position I wouldn't believe you. I love the way my life has turned out and I am so grateful for every blessing I have seen.

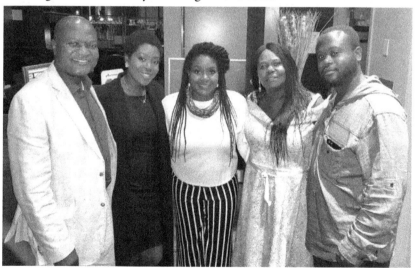

CHAPTER THIRTY-ONE

LESSONS LEARNED

- God ALWAYS has a plan

- We all have access to rose coloured glasses but it's up to us to decide if we want to wear them.

- If you want something, go get it! Even if it seems impossible, out of your league or greater than your wildest dreams, that's even more reasons to go for it.

- Life is an exchange. You can't have it all. Everything you desire requires sacrifice.

- There's no such thing as perfection, do everything the best you can and if someone doesn't think it's good enough, then it was never meant for them.

- You know yourself and your body better than anyone else, no medical textbook can teach anyone to understand the experience of living in your body. So, speak up.

- Educate yourself. You are your best advocate but you need to know what's out there to advocate for it.

- You are more powerful and can endure more than you think, so never stop pushing forward. Every day is a new day, so you can choose to leave yesterday behind or drag it along like a ton of bricks.

- Only surround yourself with people, circumstances and experiences that serve you. Life is too precious to waste it.

- You're never really alone. We choose to believe that we are alone but God is always there through the good times and the bad. Lean into Him and let your worries go.

My life has been a journey that I never could have anticipated or planned for. None of this would have been possible without God. He guided me from the start and he will carry me to the end. He has given me a testimony of resilience, hope and faith. I believe when God blesses you it's important that you share with others and bless them as well.

When I was young, I wished I knew someone that had sickle cells and was achieving the goals that I aspired to one day reach. I strive to be that person for other health warriors that are searching for the strength within them to keep going. My friends thank you for coming along with me on this journey. I pray you never give up because with God anything is possible. My new life is beyond my wildest dreams, I love this life and new normal I have been creating. If there's anyone reading this that is ready to give up because it feels like their situation will never change. Remember, I was diagnosed with a life threatening disease that had a life expectancy of 14 and I am now 29 years old and counting living the life of my dreams, and 100% sickle cells free. God truly makes the impossible possible.

THE END

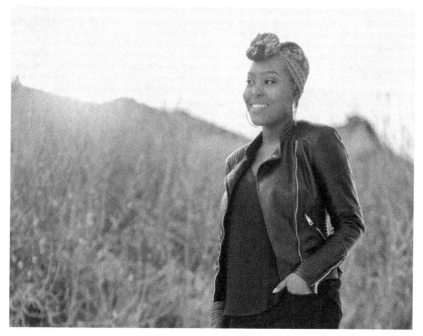

GLOSSARY

Advocate - one who pleads the cause of another https://www.merriam-webster.com/dictionary/advocate.

Apheresis/Red Cell Exchange: Apheresis is the process of withdrawing blood, filtering something out of the blood, and then putting the filtered blood back into the body. https://myhealth.alberta.ca/Health/aftercareinformation/pages/conditions.aspx-?hwid=abs2246. In my case I was getting my sickled red blood cells filtered out. My sisters stem cell collection was done through Apheresis.

Bronchoscopy: A bronchoscopy is a test that allows your doctor to examine your airways. Your doctor will thread an instrument called a bronchoscope through your nose or mouth and down your throat to reach your lungs. The bronchoscope is made of a flexible fiber-optic material and has a light source and a camera on the end https://www.healthline.com/health/bronchoscopy.

Chemotherapy: Chemotherapy is a drug treatment that uses powerful chemicals to kill fast-growing cells in your body https://www.mayoclinic.org/tests-procedures/chemotherapy/about/pac-20385033.

CRISPR: CRISPR technology is a simple yet powerful tool for editing genomes. It allows researchers to easily alter DNA sequences and modify gene function. Its many potential applications include correcting genetic defects, treating and preventing the spread of diseases and improving crops https://www.livescience.com/58790-crispr-explained.html.

Computerized Tomography (CT): A computerized tomography (CT) scan combines a series of X-ray images taken from different angles around your body and uses computer processing to create cross-sectional images (slices) of the bones, blood vessels and soft tissues inside your body https://www.mayoclinic.org/tests-procedures/ct-scan/about/pac-20393675.

Conditioning phase: The treatments used to prepare a patient for stem cell transplantation (a procedure in which a person receives blood stem cells, which make any type of blood cell). A conditioning regimen may include chemotherapy, monoclonal antibody therapy, and radiation to the entire body https://www.cancer.gov/publications/dictionaries/cancer-terms/def/conditioning-regimen.

Echocardiogram: An echocardiogram uses sound waves to produce images of your heart. This common test allows your doctor to see your heart beating and pumping blood. Your doctor can use the images from an echocardiogram to identify heart disease https://www.mayoclinic.org/tests-procedures/echocardiogram/about/pac-20393856.

Egg Freezing: Egg freezing, also known as mature oocyte cryopreservation, is a method used to save women's ability to get pregnant in the future. Eggs harvested from your ovaries are frozen unfertilized and stored for later use. A frozen egg can be thawed, combined with sperm in a lab and implanted in your uterus (in vitro fertilization) https://www.mayoclinic.org/tests-procedures/egg-freezing/about/pac-20384556.

Electrocardiogram (ECG): An electrocardiogram records the electrical signals in your heart. It's a common and painless test used to quickly detect heart problems and monitor your heart's health https://www.mayoclinic.org/tests-procedures/ekg/about/pac-20384983.

Engraftment: The cells you received on transplant day know where they belong in your body. They move through your bloodstream into your bone marrow. When these cells begin to grow and make new blood cells, it's called engraftment https://bethematch.org/patients-and-families/life-after-transplant/physical-health-and-recovery/engraftment/.

Femoral line: A femoral CVL is a soft, long, thin, flexible tube used in children who need IV medications, chemotherapy, hemodialysis, apheresis, or IV fluids. The tip of the catheter is inserted into a vein in the leg and is guided into the large vein leading to the heart https://www.aboutkidshealth.ca/article?contentid=3819&language=english.

Gallstones: Gallstones are hardened deposits of digestive fluid that can form in your gallbladder. Your gallbladder is a small, pear-shaped organ on the right side of your abdomen, just beneath your liver https://www.mayoclinic.org/diseases-conditions/gallstones/symptoms-causes/syc-20354214.

Graft Versus Host Disease (GVHD): Graft-versus-host-disease (GVHD) can happen after an allogeneic stem cell transplant. An allogeneic transplant uses stem cells from someone else (a donor) instead of your own stem cells. The stem cells from the donor develop into a new immune system that will identify and destroy cancer cells. But it can also attack your healthy cells and cause damage to tissues and organs https://www.cancer.ca/en/cancer-information/diagnosis-and-treatment/managing-side-effects/graft-versus-host-disease-gvhd/?region=on.

Granulocyte Colony Stimulating Factor (GCSF): Is used to stimulate the production of granulocytes (a type of white blood cell) in patients undergoing therapy that will cause low white blood cell counts. This medication is used to prevent infection and neutropenic (low white blood cells) fevers caused by chemotherapy http://chemocare.com/chemotherapy/drug-info/g-csf.aspx.

Immunosuppressant: Immunosuppressant drugs are a class of drugs that suppress, or reduce, the strength of the body's immune system. Some of these drugs are used to make the body less likely to reject a transplanted organ, such as a liver, heart, or kidney. These drugs are called anti-rejection drugs https://www.healthline.com/health/immunosuppressant-drugs.

Implanted Venous Access Device (IVAD): An IVAD is a small device that is surgically inserted completely beneath your skin. The IVAD is a hollow device (reservoir or port) attached to a flexible tube (catheter). The reservoir is placed beneath your skin on your chest or upper arm, and the catheter is inserted into a large vein in your chest https://vch.eduhealth.ca/media/VCH/FA/FA.200.Im7.pdf.

Intravenous (IV): Intravenous fluid regulation is the control of the amount of fluid you receive intravenously, or through your bloodstream. The fluid is given from a bag connected to an intravenous line. This is a thin tube, often called an IV, that's inserted into one of your veins https://www.healthline.com/health/intravenous-fluid-regulation.

Iron Deficiency Anemia: Iron deficiency anemia is the most common type of anemia, and it occurs when your body doesn't have enough of the mineral iron. Your body needs iron to make hemoglobin. When there isn't enough iron in your blood stream, the rest of your body can't get the amount of oxygen it needs https://www.healthline.com/health/iron-deficiency-anemia#_noHeader-PrefixedContent.

Hematologist: Hematologists are internal medicine doctors or pediatricians who have extra training in disorders related to your blood, bone marrow, and lymphatic system https://www.webmd.com/a-to-z-guides/what-is-hematologist.

Hydroxyurea: This medication is used by people with sickle cell anemia to reduce the number of painful crises caused by the disease and to reduce the need for blood transfusions. Some brands are also used to treat certain types of cancer https://www.webmd.com/drugs/2/drug-7818/hydroxyurea-oral/details.

Methemoglobinemia: Methemoglobinemia is a blood disorder in which too little oxygen is delivered to your cells. Oxygen is carried through your bloodstream by hemoglobin, a protein that's attached to your red blood cells. Normally, hemoglobin then releases that oxygen to cells throughout your body. However, there's a specific type of hemoglobin known as methemoglobin that carries oxygen through your blood but doesn't release it to the cells. If your body produces too much methemoglobin, it can begin to replace your normal hemoglobin. This can lead to not enough oxygen getting to your cells https://www.healthline.com/health/methemoglobinemia.

Narcotic: Narcotics are also called opioid pain relievers. They are only used for pain that is severe and is not helped by other types of painkillers. When used carefully and under a health care provider's direct care, these drugs can be effective at reducing pain https://medlineplus.gov/ency/article/007489.htm.

Oncologist: Oncology is the study of cancer. An oncologist is a doctor who treats cancer and provides medical care for a person diagnosed with cancer https://www.cancer.net/navigating-cancer-care/cancer-basics/cancer-care-team/types-oncologists.

Ophthalmologist: Ophthalmology is the study of medical conditions relating to the eye. Ophthalmologists are doctors who specialize in the medical and surgical treatment of this organ. A general practice doctor may refer someone to an ophthalmologist if they show symptoms of cataracts, eye infections, optic nerve problems, or other eye conditions https://www.medicalnewstoday.com/articles/326753.

Ovarian Hyper Stimulation Syndrome (OHSS): Ovarian hyperstimulation syndrome is an exaggerated response to excess hormones. It usually occurs in women taking injectable hormone medications to stimulate the development of eggs in the ovaries. Ovarian hyperstimulation syndrome (OHSS) causes the ovaries to swell and become painful https://www.mayoclinic.org/diseases-conditions/ovarian-hyperstimulation-syndrome-ohss/symptoms-causes/syc-20354697.

Peripherally Inserted Central Catheter (PICC): peripherally inserted central catheter (PICC), also called a PICC line, is a long, thin tube that's inserted through a vein in your arm and passed through to the larger veins near your heart. Very rarely, the PICC line may be placed in your leg https://www.mayoclinic.org/tests-procedures/picc-line/about/pac-20468748.

Phlebotomist: Phlebotomists take samples of blood for testing. The blood samples may be needed to learn more about a particular patient, or they may be used in research. Phlebotomists also collect blood from donors for those in need of blood transfusions https://www.webmd.com/a-to-z-guides/what-is-a-phlebotomist.

Positron Emission Tomography (PET): A positron emission tomography (PET) scan is an imaging test that allows your doctor to check for diseases in your body. The scan uses a special dye containing radioactive tracers. These tracers are either swallowed, inhaled, or injected into a vein in your arm depending on what part of the body is being examined. Certain organs and tissues then absorb the tracer https://www.healthline.com/health/pet-scan.

Pulmonary embolism: Pulmonary embolism is a blockage in one of the pulmonary arteries in your lungs. In most cases, pulmonary embolism is caused by blood clots that travel to the lungs from deep veins in the legs or, rarely, from veins in other parts of the body (deep vein thrombosis) https://www.mayoclinic.org/diseases-conditions/pulmonary-embolism/symptoms-causes/syc-20354647.

Sickle Cell Crises: A sickle cell crisis is a painful episode that may begin suddenly in a person who has sickle cell disease. A sickle cell crisis occurs when sickle shaped red blood cells clump together and block small blood vessels that carry blood to certain organs, muscles, and bones. This causes mild to severe pain. The pain can last from hours to days https://www.uofmhealth.org/health-library/hw253529.

Sickle Cell Disease: Sickle cell anemia is one of a group of disorders known as sickle cell disease. Sickle cell anemia is an inherited red blood cell disorder in which there aren't enough healthy red blood cells to carry oxygen throughout your body https://www.mayoclinic.org/diseases-conditions/sickle-cell-anemia/symptoms-causes/syc-20355876.

Total body irradiation: A type of radiation therapy that is given to the entire body. Total-body irradiation is often used with high-dose anticancer drugs to help prepare a patient for a stem cell transplant https://www.cancer.gov/publications/dictionaries/cancer-terms/def/total-body-irradiation.

X-Ray: An X-ray is a quick, painless test that produces images of the structures inside your body — particularly your bones https://www.mayoclinic.org/tests-procedures/x-ray/about/pac-20395303.

CONTACT THE AUTHOR

Revée Agyepong would like to hear from you. She can be reach on these platforms.

Website: www.reveeagyepong.com

Email: hello@mysickledcells.com

Instagram/Facebook: @mysickledcells

YouTube: mysickledcells

Address: PO Box: PO Box 83017 Webber Greens PO Edmonton, AB T5T6S1

ABOUT THE BOOK

Revée Agyepong was 12 years when she typed in the words Sickle Cell Disease into the google search bar. Her heart sank, jaw dropped and eyes swelled up with tears when she saw the life expectancy of 14 years flash across the screen. Believing she only had two years left to live she started working on a bucket list and went into survival mode. Over the years she experienced everything from crippling pain crises, pulmonary embolism scares, heavy medication therapy, high powered blood transfusions and multiple surgeries. Feeling forgotten by God, she found herself hopeless and running out of options. Revée was confused when she passed the age of 14; she truly had no idea that God had a bigger plan for her life. With the help of her sister, she pushed for an opportunity to be cured of sickle cell disease via stem cell transplant. At the time she was an adult and stem cell transplant was only an option for pediatric patients. She remained persistent and eventually her Hematologist agreed to send a referral to the transplant team. With only a 14% chance to have a donor match without sickle cell disease in her family, Revée and her entire family were overjoyed when they found that her old sister was a 10/10 perfect match! She became one of the first adult in Western Canada to undergo a stem cell transplant to cure sickle cell disease. God blessed Revée with a second chance at life and this time she gets to do it sickle cell free! Despite her challenges, she didn't allow herself to give up. She became a fierce advocate for herself and others and continues to dedicate her life to paving the way for those that follow. Come along with Revée on this triumphant story of determination, grit and the power of God.

ABOUT THE AUTHOR

Revée Agyepong is a registered nurse, health advocate and entre-preneur. She was born and raised in Edmonton, Alberta, Canada to Ghanaian parents and grew up alongside her two older siblings. Revée currently works in a pediatric hematology clinic where she has the privilege of using her personal experiences and education to empower and encourage families. In her down time, she runs a natural skin care business called Rêve Naturals and pursues oppor-tunities to raise awareness for sickle cells.